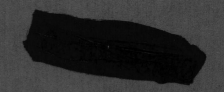

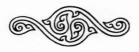

TURNING
HEALTH CARE
LEADERSHIP
AROUND

Thomas A. Atchison

TURNING HEALTH CARE LEADERSHIP AROUND

Cultivating Inspired, Empowered, and Loyal Followers

 Jossey-Bass Publishers

San Francisco • Oxford • 1990

TURNING HEALTH CARE LEADERSHIP AROUND
Cultivating Inspired, Empowered, and Loyal Followers
  by Thomas A. Atchison

Copyright © 1990 by: Jossey-Bass Inc., Publishers
                     350 Sansome Street
                     San Francisco, California 94104
                             &
                     Jossey-Bass Limited
                     Headington Hill Hall
                     Oxford OX3 0BW

Library of Congress Cataloging-in-Publication Data

Atchison, Thomas A., date.
  Turning health care leadership around.
  (The Jossey-Bass health series)
  Includes bibliographical references and index.
  1. Health services administration.   2. Hospitals—
Personnel management.   I. Title.   II. Series.
[DNLM: 1. Health Services—organization & administra-
tion. 2. Leadership. 3. Personnel Management.
W 84.1 A863t]
RA971.A88   1990   362.1′068   90-5192
ISBN 1-55542-295-0 (alk. paper)

Manufactured in the United States of America

The paper in this book meets the guidelines for
permanence and durability of the Committee on
Production Guidelines for Book Longevity of the
Council on Library Resources.

JACKET DESIGN BY WILLI BAUM

FIRST EDITION

Code 9098

The Jossey-Bass Health Series

Contents

Preface

Today's health care executives are constantly searching for ways to make their organizations more profitable, more respected, more competitive—in a word, *more effective*. But what is the essence of organizational effectiveness? Restructuring, joint ventures, and integrated health care clusters have all been seen as cures for a variety of health care's ills. But what will it really mean to be a vigorous, forward-looking health care organization in the 1990s and beyond?

Many health care executives no doubt think that environmental pressures have caused their problems. In reality, however, most of their problems result from weak leadership. Some health care organizations have yet to figure out what they are and why they exist. As a result, they communicate mixed messages to employees, physicians, trustees, and patients. This, of course, has serious consequences for the organization's human capital, as well as for the always-important bottom line.

No matter how intricate or proven its management strategy, no health care organization can be effective without inspiring its work force. It is people who carry out the mission. It is people who deliver health care services. It is people who deliver a better bottom line. Nothing, therefore, is more critical to the success of a health care organization than effective leadership of the work force. Working with over ten thousand health care professionals has reinforced my belief that health care is suffering a crisis of human capital and that leadership is the only antidote.

In many health care organizations, the staff motivation function remains exclusively focused on pay, performance appraisal, recruitment, and labor relations. In fact, however, it is the CEO who must inspire intrinsic motivation by asking such vital and provocative questions as: Why are we here? What do we believe in? Where are we headed? How can we arrive at our goals? And, most important, How do we get everyone in this organization to buy into our mission, values, and vision?

And yet these issues—mission, values, and vision—must be addressed if a health care organization is to be successful. Only through the CEO's leadership—supported by an involved board, medical staff, and management team—can a health care organization fulfill its mission and guarantee its future.

In the years ahead, we can expect a growing shortage of key personnel such as nurses, pharmacists, physical therapists, and product-line managers. Concurrently, obsolescence of other areas, such as routine diagnostic tests, low-risk inpatient birthing suites, and acute care beds, may escalate the need for effective and compassionate downsizing. The amount and speed of these changes demand that health care organizations make major investments in recruiting and retaining key professionals as well as in developing their employees. In essence, to meet the needs of a changing marketplace, health care organizations must train employees not only to meet the special needs of today's populations but also to master such areas as information systems, product-line management, sales management, and physician ventures. These are the growth areas of the future.

However, none of these changes will occur unless health care executives take the lead in shaping their corporate cultures so that the basic motivational values of employees come to match the core work values of the organization. Executives must build cultures that foster innovation, service, quality, and profitability. Incentive systems cannot do the job alone. What is needed is an inspirational leader who can create a system that allows both for downward communication of the organization's mission, values, and vision and for upward communication of results and innovation.

Traditionally, health care organizations have operated on the assumption that there are three major groups of players in the health care game: management, physicians, and trustees. There is little doubt that cooperation among these groups is more important than ever to the success of health care organizations. However, given the continually escalating demands of patients and payers, such organizations can no longer be content to focus only on constituencies and groups. Instead, they must concentrate on the primary concerns, values, and motivation of the individuals who comprise these groups.

Both for now and in the years ahead, the pivotal factors for an organization—and for all its constituencies—will be its mission, values, and vision. It is within the context of these critical issues that the central issue for the health care leader emerges: How can leadership create, mobilize, and motivate an organizational team—management, physicians, trustees, employees—to achieve an organization's vision in the context of a values-based mission?

Turning Health Care Leadership Around provides a practical, step-by-step process for assessing, mobilizing, and motivating a health care organization's work force. It focuses on how a true leader can create new ways of thinking and behaving—ways that not only will result in more productive and satisfied employees but will also help these employees achieve the organizational objectives of quality and profitability.

The book shows that health care executives become leaders by using their time, talent, and energy to understand their employees' values, perceptions, and choices. Leaders know the first step is understanding, and understanding is the first step in creating committed followers.

A personal guidebook, *Turning Health Care Leadership Around* is also a reference manual designed to be used whenever executives sense the need for organizational renewal. Unlike other management texts designed exclusively for use in the executive suite, however, this volume contains a message for everyone in the health care organization. Everyone needs to become better at dealing with the daily pressures. The best way to survive and thrive in the nineties is to reform both attitude and spirit. Everyone needs to become more interdependent, understanding, and empowering. This book shows how. The ultimate reward of the book is that it will help create a more effective health care organization—one that fulfills its mission and serves its identified markets by bringing meaning and value to the lives of all its employees.

This is a book about leadership strategies that build committed workers. It challenges health care executives to put as much emphasis on motivation and commitment as on profitability and strategy. I try to demonstrate how leadership that balances both sets of concerns differs from the usual kind of leadership that emphasizes profitability and strategy, and I refer to these concerns as the tangible and intangible elements of the organization.

The book uses Maehr and Braskamp's *The Motivation Factor: A Theory of Personal Investment* (1986) to review the intangible elements of an organization. The premise of my book is that the tangible aspects of leadership—cash flow, market share, productivity, policy and procedures, and so on—are important and must be attended to but that the intangibles—culture, mission, and values— must also be understood and developed. Each chapter explores how to cultivate these intangible aspects in hands-on, practical ways and uses exercises and examples to aid readers in applying the skills.

The book acknowledges how the onset of prospective payment redirected the attention of health care executives. An industrywide shock occurred when the government and later insurance companies began to pay hospitals a fixed price. For twenty-five years prior to 1984, hospitals were not run by businesses. There were few incentives to produce the best value. The era before diagnosis-related groups (DRGs) can be characterized as "more is better." This all changed when cost control began to determine a hospital's economic viability. Now that cost systems are firmly in place, the effects of economics on health care professionals must be dealt with. Health care executives have begun to place more emphasis on financial than on human capital. This book addresses the need to get a high return on human capital. It calls for a rethinking of health care leadership in the 1990s by focusing on how to create committed followers.

Overview of the Contents

Part One introduces readers to the language of health care intangibles and the impact that these intangibles can have on organizational effectiveness.

Chapter One challenges the reader to face the changing realities of health care. It studies the role of the leader in a changing environment. The chapter discusses various kinds of leaders and explores the differences in their styles. It says that leaders create followers and that they do so by building a living corporate culture. Health care leaders are challenged to take on a new set of behaviors that will unleash the potential of the work force in the context of the corporate culture.

Chapter Two highlights and challenges a variety of myths concerning mission, motivation, and management. Through examples, the chapter demonstrates that change cannot occur in organizations that find themselves under the spell of these myths. It also defines the change process and spells out some of the problems that will come with its implementation. Finally, it provides guidelines for effecting change.

Chapter Three answers the question, Why do people work? The book uses *The Motivation Factor: A Theory of Personal Investment* to define how motivation works toward commitment. By confirming that all people are motivated all the time, it answers the argument that some workers cannot be motivated. Chapter Three suggests that you watch how people spend their time, talent, and energy, and it argues that worker motivation is based on four dominant values: recognition, accomplishment, power, and affiliation. It explores how these values are demonstrated in the health care environment and in decision making.

Chapter Four discusses in more detail how motivation works. It tells the reader to look at the personalities of employees, the characteristics of their jobs, and the culture of the organization in which the employees work. A strong corporate culture, where all understand the values and their role in demonstrating those values, is the key to managing change. The techniques to measure and manage change are becoming very important as the pressures on health care continue. This chapter emphasizes the adjustments that health care organizations will continue to experience and makes clear that job satisfaction and commitment result from a strong match between the person, the job, and the organization. The chapter concludes by exploring how an organization's culture can be strengthened.

Part Two defines the organizational development approach to effective managed change.

Chapter Five introduces three essential change elements: assessment, analysis, and action. The chapter provides a battery of questions that readers can use to determine their perceptions of change elements and prepares them for further exploration of these elements. It is the first of four chapters that deal with assessment, analysis, and action in detail. It explores the purpose of assessments and the possible problems involved in their use, and it challenges leaders to take action and accept responsibility for assessment needs.

Chapter Six gives readers practical advice on conducting a survey. By means of questions from a health care assessment survey designed by MetriTech, Inc., readers are given the opportunity to do their own personal assessment. Having finished this chapter, readers will know what steps to take to make sure that assessment will be a positive experience for themselves and their organization.

Chapter Seven explores how leaders pass judgment on the data and make decisions accordingly once the assessment has been completed. The reader has an opportunity to look at a variety of audits, as well as possible interpretations of them. This chapter also assists the reader in identifying the values measured in each audit, and it analytically defines the relationship of the scores to their apparent meanings. Through exercises, it moves the readers from examining facts and numbers to looking at their own core values and their personal leadership styles. This chapter also shows readers how to create a meaningful vision statement.

Chapter Eight guides readers through the practical steps needed to implement a change process. Most important, it tells them whose responsibility it is to see that realistic actions are taken. A series of questions encourages readers to look at their own essential change elements and shows how to translate them into specific change behaviors. Strategies for implementing effective organizational change are outlined.

Part Three assists the reader in pulling together essential change elements and building teams into one understandable whole.

Chapter Nine addresses the issues that leaders must face during the change process: conflict resolution, role modeling, and communication. It looks at the different ways change enters an organization and offers practical methods for handling each situation. For example, traumatic change must be approached differently from developmental change; each calls for a different leadership style. This chapter offers helpful hints about the responsibilities of leaders in team building, and it draws parallels between developing an organizational team and developing an athletic team.

Chapter Ten discusses the key issues involved in producing committed followers: building business plans and unit plans, developing staff, and creating performance evaluation systems. Throughout the discussion, readers are reminded that management development is meaningless unless it is driven by the mission, values, and vision of the organization. This chapter summarizes for the reader the key message of the book: If the tangible and intangible elements of an organization are not in balance, the organization will suffer. It challenges readers to take on the new leadership roles they need to play and places the task before them: turning health care leadership around to look at the people who must be motivated.

Acknowledgments

I could not have written this book without the help of numerous friends and colleagues, each of whom had a special role and contributed his or her bit of excellence to the text. The main role was played by Alis Valencia, former health editor at Jossey-Bass. It was her confidence in the value of this undertaking and gentle but firm prodding that made it possible for me to complete this work. Other significant contributors include Nancy Davis, Joyce Flory, Marcella Hollinger, Joyce Hosty, Rebecca McGovern, and Ann Spiers.

The empirical work of Larry Braskamp and Martin Maehr provided the initial inspiration for my approach to health care leadership. In addition, Samuel Krug, president of MetriTech, Inc., produced much of the data needed for this book with his superb survey and analysis work.

I want to thank the health care leaders mentioned in the text for their assistance: Sister Alfreda Bracht, Frederick Brown, Robert Fanning, Jeffrey Norman, and Arthur Sturm. Included in spirit is Bud Atchison—leader, teacher, father.

Special thanks to Michael Bice and Kimberly Smith for using part of their Christmas holidays to review the initial draft.

Finally, Margaret Atchison deserves my gratitude for her emotional and intellectual support.

Glen Ellyn, Illinois   Thomas A. Atchison
August 1990

The Author

Thomas A. Atchison is president and founder of The Atchison Consulting Group, Inc., which specializes in organizational development. He received his B.A. degree (1967) from Northern Illinois University in psychology and his M.A. degree (1969) from Northeastern Illinois State University in special education. He received his Ed.D. degree (1977) from Loyola University of Chicago in curriculum and human resource development.

Since 1984, Atchison has consulted extensively with health care organizations, from a fifty-five–bed hospital to a $4 billion health care delivery system, on managed change programs, team building, and leadership development. He also has consulted with health care vendors and government agencies on the intangible aspects of health care. In conjunction with MetriTech, Inc., Champaign, Illinois, he developed the Healthcare Organizational Assessment Survey, a quantitative diagnostic tool used to assess the culture of health care organizations. A dynamic speaker, he has given presentations to over ten thousand health care professionals on leadership, strengthening corporate culture, the dynamics of a managed change process, employee motivation, and other elements of effective organizations. He has been a member of the Formation Committee of the Catholic Healthcare Association and is currently on the panel of advisers for the Leadership Center of the Healthcare

Forum in San Francisco. Also, he has written or been featured in a number of articles about motivation, managed change, team building, and leadership.

Atchison's expertise in health care is built on fifteen years of experience in a variety of management positions in health care institutions and organizations, such as Schwab Rehabilitation Hospital and Rush-Presbyterian-St. Luke's Medical Center, both in Chicago, as well as the American Hospital Association and the American College of Healthcare Executives.

TURNING
HEALTH CARE
LEADERSHIP
AROUND

PART ONE

The
New Leadership
Mandate

Chapter One

Changing Health Care Organizations:
The Leadership Difference

Leaders have followers. Being called the CEO and standing in front of a group does not in itself make you a leader. Without committed followers, you have nothing but a title. No matter how elegant your diversification strategy, how sophisticated your technology or how strong your financial base, you will never build an effective organization unless you can inspire others to follow your vision. The commitment of your work force must be consistently high across groups: executives, managers, supervisors, physicians, and all other employees.

Health care executives can create new services, negotiate joint ventures, and build new alliances and still be little more than bean counters and management mechanics. It is in the attitudes of their followers that we find the differences between titled executives and leaders. Management-driven executives fix problems. Leaders inspire others to achieve the organization's vision in the context of a values-based mission.

Leaders stand out. Through the force of their presence, they model why and how everyone must be committed to the organization. In today's environment, commitment among the work force is increasingly difficult to build and sustain. As they struggle to find new models of leadership, health care executives are the essence of the solution as well as part of the problem. Bruised and battered by a changing environment, many health care executives regress into rigid, autocratic management behaviors that are founded on archaic myths about people and organizations. If health care executives are to bring about change in their organizations, they must shed these myths and reject counterproductive behaviors. They must create a culture that produces lasting effects on followers by building commitment.

What do Sister Alfreda Bracht, Arthur Sturm, Robert Fanning, Jeffrey Norman, and Frederick Brown have in common? Leadership. Committed followers. In the following pages, you will see that although the organizations they head may have different structures, management styles, and priorities, all these leaders know how to build commitment to a vision. They understand the power of the intangible elements of leadership. Each possesses the essential leadership traits of intelligence, discipline, energy, and compassion. Regardless of how they express these traits, they all use them to build effective organizations.

All health care executives must now cope with rising expectations and increasing stress. To avoid being caught in the undertow, leaders monitor the organization's pulse, interact with employees, and create a corporate culture upon which to build the organization's future. The current crisis in health care leadership is not simple. It is a crisis that hinges on the delicate and critical issues of values and meaning: Who are we—really? What are we doing here? Does any of this matter? Are we making a difference in peoples' lives? In short, health care executives must reassess their role, function, and scope in today's health care environment.

From Compassion to Capitalism

Health care management is a profession without a secure context. Health care executives receive confused signals about who they are and what they should do. No one can function in a vacuum, and few people can function within a context that provides muddled or confusing messages. Yet this is what health care executives are now compelled to do.

It is part of a pattern of responses we begin to develop in childhood. From birth, we learn to respond appropriately to stimuli. When we see a red light, we stop; when we see a green light, we move. And when we enter a new setting, certain stimuli prompt or cue our behavior. If we walk into a church, for example, we become quiet, but if we walk into a football stadium, we have permission to yell and cheer. It is the context that makes behavior appropriate or inappropriate. If someone behaved in church as if it were a football stadium or showed up in a witch's costume on December 25th, that person would be labeled deviant or crazy. He would be acting out of context.

Health care executives face a similar situation. Many men and women chose health care as a profession because they felt confident and secure that, no matter what their function, they would work in a context of caring and compassion. In 1984, the prospective payment system (PPS) changed the rules and transformed the context of health care. Executives who had once worked in the altruistic context of service to the community now had to concern themselves with market share, downsizing, consolidation, and diversification. "You can heal," they were told, "but you must do it in the context of economic constraints."

Imagine the effect on their emotions and behavior. Executives began to question their attitudes, beliefs, roles and management styles and to wonder why they ever entered the profession. Wait a minute, many an executive said to himself, if I wanted to be a money-hungry businessman or a capitalist, I would never have chosen this profession.

Where changes in context occur, several patterns of reaction emerge:

> *Regression:* Insecure and afraid of the change in context, people cling to tradition and revert to nostalgic discussions of "the good old days."
>
> *Aggression:* Angry and frustrated by the change in context, people lash out at everything that represents the new order. They refuse to cooperate and even resort to sabotage.
>
> *Passivity:* Confused by the change in context, people may tolerate new initiatives but remain suspicious and detached from the process.
>
> *Symbolism:* Baffled by the change in context, people develop

an almost neurotic obsession with making symbolic gestures. Having appointed a committee or task force, they
congratulate themselves for being responsive.

Grouping: Alienated and isolated by the change in context,
people turn to others for support, encouragement, and
protection. "It's us against them," they reassure their
associates.

Leadership: Challenged by the change in context, these rare
individuals give the new context meaning and make new
rules that are understandable to the work force. This is
what is going on and this is what it means for us, they tell
their people. And here is how we can turn this change into
an opportunity to create an even more effective organization.

Sister Alfreda Bracht is such a leader. As CEO of St. Francis
Hospital in Evanston, Illinois, for over twenty-five years, Sister Alfreda has anchored her leadership by means of five core corporate
values (the Franciscan Standards): (1) Respect life; (2) be proud and
loyal to the hospital family; (3) demonstrate concern for the patient,
especially the poor, aged, and neglected; (4) show compassion, respect, and joy; and (5) carefully allocate resources and adhere to the
teachings of the Catholic Church. Her faithfulness to these standards is the essence of Sister Alfreda's success as a leader.

Therein lies the most significant difference between managers and leaders. Managers will respond to a change in context by
developing tools and gadgets to fix specific problems. They will
read books on high-performance organizations and rigidly practice
"executive rituals" to project an attitude of dynamism and credibil-
ity. Caught in the grip of their own illusions, they assume that if
they act and dress like leaders, they will be leaders. However, as in
Sister Alfreda's case, true leaders dress themselves with the corporate
values.

Ineffective organizations have little or no employee commitment because they have no anchor: no values, no belief system, no
central principle to help employees make sense of their jobs. The
employees find themselves trying to function in a confused and
disorienting context. Keeping busy is a theme in many health care

organizations, but often it is activity without purpose or meaning. In contrast, leaders address and massage the context. They show the work force how to cross the bridge from the past to the present and then explain how everyone can play a part in building yet another bridge to the future. They embrace the anxiety, frustration, and uncertainty of the work force and turn fear of change into confidence about the future.

Traps That Leaders Avoid

Health care executives may acknowledge that health care is no longer a comfortable or predictable field, but few have yet realized that leadership is the solution to their difficulties. Most remain managers with an exclusive focus on content. They create tools and techniques to make sense out of the latest crisis. Challenged by constant change and escalating demands, they become tyrannized by day-to-day problems. And, like the sirens of Ulysses, problems come to have a mysterious and seductive power over people. Unfortunately, like the sailors in ancient Greek mythology, health care executives can easily end up on the rocks—dazed and bewildered by their loss of control.

When health care executives become seduced by problems, they respond in several ways.

The Detail Trap. For some, data and detail assume the power of a religion; in meetings, these executives are often overheard saying, "We're still analyzing the data. Until we understand them, we can't really move ahead." Unresponsive to the frustration of managers, some view an obsession with fine print as the mark of a serious and tough-minded executive. The resultant "analysis paralysis" cripples progress. It permits an executive to live in a safe, no-lose world where blame for any problem rests with those who pushed for a decision before the data were analyzed completely.

The Totality Trap. Other executives move to the opposite extreme. Seduced by the magic of cosmic, macro thinking, they tell their subordinates, "I'm studying the issue; I can't decide until I understand the totality of the impact." This approach also leads to paralysis since the future can never be defined clearly enough for a commitment to be made. Both these first two types cannot be trapped in blame; they always have an out because solutions depend on an unanticipated change in the future.

   The Micro/Macro Trap. Not content with a single world-view, some executives alternate between atomic particles and the Milky Way. On Monday, this kind of executive might say to the director of planning and marketing, "This is a great idea, but give me the details. I need to see the numbers. Where are your month-by-month pro formas?" Eager to move toward a final decision, the director returns with the numbers on Friday, only to hear, "OK, now can you help me see the big picture? I want to know where this is going in the next five years." The security of a stress-reduced world has been assured because whatever position is taken, the counter position can also be taken.

   Consider the effect of these traps on executives. Rather than asking, What is the best decision for this organization? they are more apt to think, Be ready to defend against a mistake! Ultimately, employees grow weary of this retrogressive game and begin to reduce their own productivity.

   Why do health care executives run their staffs through rat mazes like these? Perhaps they feel impotent in the face of issues such as quality, financial risk, competition, managed care, and other components of today's health care trademark—*accelerated change.* Reeling from changes in regulations and reimbursement that never seem to abate, they choose a different course: securing power over people and information within the organization. With this strategy, they can control their managers with minutiae and lock their boards into a permanent holding pattern with macro thinking.

   Moving within or between the traps of detail and macro thinking, health care executives find it difficult to build commitment among their staffs. But sooner or later, the board chairperson, the president of the medical staff, or even a competitor will unveil the truth. The executives have accomplished very little because they failed to gain the support and commitment of those who did the work. They thought they were leading, but no one was following.

Other health care executives complain that they don't have time to make changes or pursue new opportunities because they have so much to do, which is yet another kind of trap.

The Checklist Trap. Some executives might want to look at how physicians are changing their practice patterns and recognize the importance of sharpening the organization's information systems' capabilities for risk-management contracts. Instead, we hear the response, "I'd like to get to those issues, but I've got so much to do. I'"m so busy right now. Things will probably get better in the spring. The timing isn't right."

Sound familiar? True, health care executives are busy professionals and their responsibilities are increasing. Being human, health care executives prefer to invest their time in tasks for which they have a good track record. If their financial reports receive rave reviews from the board, they will continue to churn them out. Some health care executives still operate on the assumption that to be important they must have a multitude of things to do. The more cluttered the calendar, the more pressing the deadlines, the more important they feel. What if, in the best of all possible worlds, they could rid themselves of their "to do" lists? Would they really be better off? Probably not. Given their assumptions about the nature of good management, they would probably invent new and different things to do.

Managers perform tasks and execute procedures. But leaders clarify and model the corporate culture so that the work force understands not only how to act but why it should act in certain ways. *Leaders give jobs meaning— a context.* And they inspire people to follow them!

For example, look at your calendar for the previous week and answer these questions:

1. How much time did you spend solving problems or crises?
2. How much time did you spend addressing issues of finance?
3. Compare the time you invested in solving problems and discussing finance with the time you invested in two other areas: communicating the mission, vision, and values of the organi-

zation and working directly with people to clarify their roles in creating a more effective organization.

Take an inventory of your phone calls for a one-week period and answer these questions:

1. What was the content and length of the phone calls you answered first?
2. What phone calls were postponed, delegated, or ignored?

Based on your analysis of both your calendar and your phone calls, what conclusions can you reach about your investment in human capital versus financial capital? How do you cope with problems involving the organization's mission, values, and vision? To what extent are you a victim of the traps of detail, totality, and micro/macro thinking? What have been the consequences for your career and for your organization? Is your job at risk because the trustees or physicians are not happy with the direction of the hospital? Have followers increased their commitment because of how you used your time, talent, and energy? If yes, congratulations. If no, read on.

Not surprisingly, there is an inverse relationship between the length of an executive's "to do" list and the effectiveness of the organization. Effective leaders have short checklists, but the people who work for them have very long checklists.

Know Where You Are Going

Executives who lead understand a critical concept: To be effective—to help their organization achieve its vision—they must work with and through people. To use the analogy developed by noted management theorist Peter Drucker, they accept their role as symphony conductor and allow competent and well-trained musicians to play the instruments. Leaders know why they are there: to inspire. They select and communicate the musical score—always making sure, of course, that their musicians are skilled enough to handle the music.

Leaders have come to another realization as well: They can

no longer simply try to solve problems as they arise. Such a process is akin to driving a car 100 miles per hour while looking through the rearview mirror. Let managers worry about the present and the immediate past; leaders must look down the road, always setting the direction by communicating their vision of the organization.

Unfortunately, health care executives have more to cope with than their own biases and assumptions about proper executive behavior. They must also confront the cataclysmic changes that have rocked the profession and industry since the early 1980s. Revenue margins have dropped, access to capital is limited, delivery of services is moving from inpatient to outpatient settings, and manpower pools are shrinking. And these are only a few of the consequences of a fundamental shift in how hospitals do their business and health care executives perform their jobs.

Like individuals, industries can suffer strokes. With the introduction in 1984 of Medicare prospective payment legislation, the health care industry suffered a stroke whose effects rippled through every hospital in America and changed the priorities and practices of the executives who manage them. As with a patient who suffers a stroke, the health care industry has had to undergo a long process of acute care and rehabilitation. Prospective payment forced executives to learn how to perform their jobs in new and different ways. Some professionals were traumatized and paralyzed by the event. Some have never recovered their ability to function, and to this day they continue to yearn for a return to a simpler time.

While some of these executives lost their positions or moved into retirement or second careers, even those who are currently at the helm of health care organizations seldom feel confident and secure. Instead, they candidly, but privately, describe themselves as threatened, frightened, angry, and confused about their profession and their careers. These are their questions and doubts:

"This isn't what I got into the health care profession for. What am I doing here?" Brought up a Catholic on the south side of Chicago, this executive once thought he would become a priest but eventually chose to put his faith into practice in a Catholic health care organization. Five years after the passage of prospective payment legislation, he concluded, "I'm going to quit this Catholic organization and go work for a Christian one." The organization was Catholic in name only. The values and traditions of hundreds of years had been eroded by an almost Machiavellian approach to business.

Others face a similar crisis in values. Some, after years in the not-for-profit sector, are lured to a dream job with a prominent investor-owned health care system. Although no one ever said it directly, these newly hired executives are expected to forget or at least downplay the values of compassion and respect for the individual in favor of increasing net shareholder value. Once they realize this, they must leave if they are to keep mind and soul intact.

"What next?" Most people find it difficult to accept the continuing acceleration of change, and health care executives are no exception to this rule. Many are growing increasingly insecure about their ability to predict the future and wonder what new dragon might be lurking around the corner. Among their questions: What will be the next constituency to challenge, monitor, or even try to police the health care system? Will it be government, payers, business, or providers themselves? What new demands will these groups make? What strains will the aging of the population place on resources? Will it require a retooling of the health care system? Armed with data on providers and outcomes, how far will consumers go in pushing for changes from physicians and hospitals? Will greater involvement from the business community mean even higher demands for accurate data, cost management, and quality of care? Finally, will the escalating costs of technology mean lower quality of care and even denial of care for some patients?

"What does it all mean for me?" As leaders scan the environment, they try to analyze, interpret, and evaluate what these trends will mean for their organizations. They must bring the trends home to the minds and hearts of the workers. Exhibit 1 is an exercise that can help to envision the future.

Dealing with Uncertainty

"Will my organization survive?" Environmental assessments and studies of the future show a decided lack of confidence in the future. Supported by hard statistics on hospital bed occupancy and revenue margins, experts predict that the movement toward outpatient care will continue to threaten the profitability and cash flow

Exhibit 1. Looking to the Future.

Directions: Write a short statement about where your organization will stand on each issue twenty-four months from now.

Growing Consumer Clout: How are we going to differentiate our services to attract new patients and retain old ones? What kinds of services can be developed to attract our senior population?

In twenty-four months we will _____

_____

Access: How can we do our part in addressing the indigent care problem in this community given our lower operating surpluses?

In twenty-four months we will _____

_____

Physician/Hospital Relationship: How can we help our physicians with their practices and make them partners in the success of this organization?

In twenty-four months we will _____

_____

Pressures from Payers: How can we promote direct contracting with employers and give them the cost and utilization data they want?

In twenty-four months we will _____

_____

Financial Risk: What alternative forms of financing are available? How can we reevaluate programs to cut unnecessary expenses?

In twenty-four months we will _____

_____

Quality: What does quality mean to the people in this community, and how do we get everyone in this organization to buy into the concept? How can we make quality part of the way we deliver care and do business?

In twenty-four months we will _____

_____

Technology: How do we evaluate the purchase of life-saving technology when the government has yet to approve payment?

In twenty-four months we will _____

_____

of hospitals. On a personal level, executives—especially those who head troubled inner-city or rural institutions—fight to revive organizations brought down by forces beyond their control.

"Am I going to be here next year?" The turnover of health care executives increased, according to a national survey, from 7.5 percent in 1981 to 16.5 percent in 1987. The bleak message in these numbers is reinforced by painful stories of forced terminations:

- A CEO returns from an annual meeting to find that his desk has been cleaned out and another individual is already sitting in his chair.
- A parent board appoints an attorney as its hatchet man, and he tells the CEO, "Look, because of philosophical differences the board has decided you're going and that's all there is to it. Let's see if we can work something out in terms of your future."
- A CEO attends a conference in another city with two of his board members. He receives a call telling him that other board members have voted him out of his job.
- A CEO is compelled by financial pressures to recommend shutting down the hospital. Influential doctors get to the board chairman. The conclusion: Time for a change in leadership. The CEO leaves.
- An executive is brought in to run a medical equipment business, but the holding company withdraws its support after six months. After having relocated from another state, the executive is out of a job.
- Throughout the country, entire marketing and other staff departments find themselves being phased out as organizations begin to question the cost and value of these functions.

"I've got a thirty-year mortgage and a two-year job," confessed one health care executive. Others who were once secure in their positions now wonder, Could it happen to me? The answer is yes. Most executives lose jobs not because of incompetence, but because of more elusive factors such as fit, chemistry, or personality. Forced termination is now a widely accepted risk in executive ranks.

Executives must learn to focus on leadership skills such as inspiring workers, clarifying values, and visioning. Unfortunately, many executives are adrift in a sea of diagnostic tests, workbooks and seminars that are often geared to other industries and to younger professionals.

Executives can usually accept loneliness at the top if they have a network of colleagues with whom they can share ideas and resources. In years past, health care executives routinely reported on shared plans for new programs and services with CEOs of neighboring hospitals, but they no longer do so. The interaction among executives of rival institutions at business meetings and social events may be polite, but it is rarely friendly. If executives want a professional sounding board, they must seek out their counterparts in noncompeting markets and even in other industries.

Suspicion and mistrust extend to other areas of the organization as well. Health care executives routinely report stories of physicians who admit to four different hospitals and of nurses who—without reservation—walk down the street to take a job with a competitor. Physicians review building plans for a new diagnostic imaging center at a board meeting and then proceed to build the center themselves—on the same site chosen by the hospital.

Betrayal is even more painful when health care executives have invested time in mentoring a fledgling manager. "There is no loyalty among management staff today," confessed one discouraged administrator. "You can mentor a kid, promote her in the organization, and she can go down the street and take your strategic plan with her."

The urgency to move up and out as quickly as possible may reflect the values of a generation mesmerized by quarterly earnings, MBA degrees, and "power suits." But this is small consolation to health care executives. Without a loyal and committed work force—managers, physicians, nurses, and board members—an effective organization cannot be built.

The hospital is no longer simply the big white building down the street. Instead, it is a health care delivery continuum that must balance outpatient care, diagnostic treatment, inpatient care, and rehabilitation with changing market requirements and the need to find new sources of revenue. Despite these trends, however, physicians, trustees, and community leaders often challenge executives who are trying to diversify services. Out of tradition or self-preservation some want to transform the big white building into a permanent community shrine. They often refuse to see the relevance of women's health centers, industrial medicine programs, sports medicine clinics, and clinical laboratories because they believe these conflict with the hospital's basic mission of taking care of the acutely ill.

However, health care executives are very aware that operating margins are shrinking, and they know they can never replicate past growth in hospital-based acute care. The bed is dead! Their only salvation is to create a culture that encourages development of profitable niches—from pain clinics to centers dedicated to diagnostic imaging, treatment of cancer, birthing, and hospice care.

"Some of my employees think I'm out of touch. Don't they know what I'm trying to do?" Health care leaders must think at least five years out, addressing issues such as: How are we going to diversify? Which competitors should we worry about? But managers want new equipment right now and show little patience when an executive replies, "You don't understand; we've got to consider where we will be five years out. Managers and physicians have been known to retort, "Forget five years. We've got people sitting in the hallways and we can't find beds for them." Fresh from twelve-hour shifts, these beleaguered employees frequently conclude, "If he doesn't care about these patients, then why should we care about them? We might as well look for jobs down the street."

"Why are we here? What's our mission? What do we mean to this community?" Health care leaders must question their organizational identity: "Are we a community service? Or are we just a machine to make money? And how do I balance charity, compassion, and caring with the need for profitability through diversification and cost cutting?"

Closer to home, employees question mission statements that consist of lofty platitudes. What happens when community members see slick hospital advertisements that indicate the hospital is in hot pursuit of a new market segment? And what happens to commitment when employees hear nothing but reports on business structures, marketing strategies, and information systems aimed at creating a more businesslike atmosphere?

Leaders inspire followers to do things faster and better. For years, health care executives used a command/control management style and employed relatively long decision cycles. Now, however, this approach is more likely to lose opportunities than to win them. Although executives may want to become more democratic and participatory, they sometimes lack the skills, confidence, and experience to do so. They may want a flatter organization, but their inner voice murmurs, Be careful of everything and make sure decisions are *perfect*. Some health care executives cope by shifting into neutral and coasting the rest of the way. "All I've got to do is tough this out until age fifty-nine and a half," confessed one CEO with only five years to go. "Then I can collect my pension."

What health care executives are now experiencing is nothing short of a collapse of the old order. The rules that worked for so many years no longer work. Today's health care leaders must master a new set of behaviors if they are to unleash the potential of the work force within the context of the corporate culture.

Chapter Two

Bridging
Myth and Reality

Strengthening the corporate culture takes a big commitment from everyone in the organization. Because we are creatures of habit, we tend to be uneasy about changes, particularly big changes. We start to look for reasons to resist change. In doing so, we practice such "arts" as avoiding the facts, setting up obstacles, and using false arguments and generalizations.

Starting to Manage Change

Being aware of and prepared for resistance is the first step in overcoming it. This chapter reviews some typical myths that people use to justify resistance to a culture enhancement process and debunks these myths.

Myths of Mission

1. *"We need a mission that protects our not-for-profit status, so let the lawyers write it."* Protecting a not-for-profit status is a noble goal, but it may have little or nothing to do with the organization's mission, that is, with its reason for existence. A self-protective statement drafted by attorneys will do nothing to enhance commitment, motivate staff, or help employees focus on vision.

2. *"Mission statements are for the community, not for management."* A mission statement answers one important question: Why does this organization exist? Unless health care executives know and understand their purpose, they will find themselves trapped in defensive positions. While a mission statement may have various impacts on external audiences, it is not really written for the community. Of course, community leaders may read the mission statement, and the statement may even change their image of the organization. But in contrast to physicians, trustees, employees, and managers, community residents will never live the mission in their daily lives.

3. *"Mission statements should be lofty, eloquent, and long."* Mission statements should not contain more than three or four basic ideas, and these ideas should be easy to remember. They should be expressed skillfully, but in "plain speak" and in short, tight sentences. The best mission statements distill the essence of the organization.

4. *"Mission statements must be idealistic."* If mission statements are idealistic, they become ineffective. Instead, the mission statement should define in very specific terms why the organization exists. Although the statement may incorporate such value-laden words as *charity* and *healing*, the work force must see a close connection between the language of the statement and what they do on the job. They must understand how they make the organization's mission come alive.

5. *"Mission statements are worthless. They have little practical value in day-to-day management."* If mission statements are idealistic and impractical, they are indeed worthless. When the mission statement focuses on an organization's real reason for existence, however, it becomes the acid test for all decisions: hiring, formulating budgets, expanding operations, downsizing, and adding new services.

The classic example of a mission statement is Johnson & Johnson's credo (Exhibit 2). While the Johnson & Johnson credo is lengthy, it defines the four reasons why the company exists: responsibility to doctors, nurses, patients, and mothers; responsibility to employees; responsibility to communities; and respon-

Exhibit 2. Johnson & Johnson Credo.

Our Credo

We believe our first responsibility is to the doctors, nurses and patients,
to mothers and fathers and all others who use our products and services.
In meeting their needs everything we do must be of high quality.
We must constantly strive to reduce our costs
in order to maintain reasonable prices.
Customers' orders must be serviced promptly and accurately.
Our suppliers and distributors must have an opportunity
to make a fair profit.

We are responsible to our employees,
the men and women who work with us throughout the world.
Everyone must be considered as an individual.
We must respect their dignity and recognize their merit.
They must have a sense of security in their jobs.
Compensation must be fair and adequate,
and working conditions clean, orderly and safe.
We must be mindful of ways to help our employees fulfill
their family responsibilities.
Employees must feel free to make suggestions and complaints.
There must be equal opportunity for employment, development
and advancement for those qualified.
We must provide competent management,
and their actions must be just and ethical.

We are responsible to the communities in which we live and work
and to the world community as well.
We must be good citizens — support good works and charities
and bear our fair share of taxes.
We must encourage civic improvements and better health and education.
We must maintain in good order
the property we are privileged to use,
protecting the environment and natural resources.

Our final responsibility is to our stockholders.
Business must make a sound profit.
We must experiment with new ideas.
Research must be carried on, innovative programs developed
and mistakes paid for.
New equipment must be purchased, new facilities provided
and new products launched.
Reserves must be created to provide for adverse times.
When we operate according to these principles,
the stockholders should realize a fair return.

Johnson & Johnson

Source: Reprinted with permission of Johnson & Johnson.

sibility to stockholders. In addition, it includes Johnson & Johnson's corporate values:

Quality	Equal opportunity
Reasonable prices	Competence
Customer service	Justice
Fair profit	Ethics
Dignity of the individual	Citizenship
Security	Innovation
Fairness	Responsibility
Openness	Prudence

When the Tylenol crisis hit, there was no question about the action that Johnson & Johnson would take. Their mission statement gave them no alternative but to remove the product from the shelves.

6. *"Why bother with a mission statement? Employees never understand mission statements anyway."* It is true that, in the past, mission statements were often misunderstood by everyone in the organization, including executives and trustees. But if executives properly communicate the mission, every employee in the organization—from the board chairperson to the nurse's aide—will understand the statement and be able to apply it to job performance.

7. *"Trustees can't function without traditional mission statements."* Trustees have generally preferred long and lofty mission statements that celebrated the organization's traditions and history—and some still maintain that bias. As a result, many organizations now supplement their mission statements with statements that set forth their philosophy, standards, or principles. These statements should echo the organization's core values.

The ideal mission statement, however, should be clear and direct: "We exist to provide a continuum of high-quality care to the residents of our community." In addition, the mission statement should be used as the first criterion or standard for making decisions. On the one hand, if an organization exists to provide a continuum of high-quality care to community residents, it would resist investments in regional medical care programs. On the other hand, it might pursue opportunities in home care, long-term care, or women's health.

Many mission statements incorporate the organization's core values. These values are the convictions that drive all behavior, and it is only when the core corporate values and the fundamental personal values of the employees come together that strong commitment emerges. Without solid grounding in a values-based mission, employees may fulfill job requirements, but they will do little to make the organization more effective. When staff members function outside the context of the values-based mission, they may or may not support the organization. Their primary goal may be simply to do their job and get a paycheck.

As there are myths of mission, so there are myths of motivation—myths grounded in misperceptions of human nature and how people work and function. In confronting and exploding these myths, health care leaders should look within to ascertain what personal traits, experiences, or attitudes are holding them back so they must rely on these myths as crutches.

Myths of Motivation

1. *"Most employees are motivated by money."* The reality is that most employees are motivated by personal feelings of self-worth. In some organizations, however, the only way employees receive recognition is through their paychecks. But money has its limitations. Money functions as an incentive on only one level, and it is a disincentive on two others. Money is an incentive when it fits employees' perception of their worth. However, if compensation is too low, employees will feel used. At the same time, if compensation is far beyond the position's market value, employees will fear that they may lose their jobs if they are ever "discovered." In addition, their sense of self-esteem will inevitably erode if they feel they are not earning what they are being paid.

In general, the motivational effect of financial compensation is related inversely to the respect that employees receive. The more employees are mistreated or ignored, the more they demand higher pay. This relationship between respect and money is one of the most misunderstood causes of ineffectiveness in health care organizations.

2. *"Some people can't be motivated."* The reality is that everyone is 100 percent motivated 100 percent of the time. Everyone has a full reservoir of motivation. The caveat is that people may not be motivated to do what the organization wants them to do. A nurse, for example, may be highly motivated to organize her unit, socialize with other nurses, or pick arguments with physicians. In contrast, a dietician may be motivated to do very little because of a lack of incentives. If I try something new, I'll get yelled at, she concludes. But if I maintain the status quo, my manager will leave me alone. In the same way, an admitting clerk will glance at his paycheck and conclude, "If I work really hard, I will get a 3 percent raise. But if I continue working at the same pace, I will probably still get a 3 percent raise." The lesson is clear: If rewards and recognition are scarce, employees typically see no reason to alter or enhance their behavior. Unfortunately, the executive may conclude, Staff members aren't motivated to do new things; they're not risk takers. The reality is that the employees may be risk takers who are trapped in an organization that offers no reasons for taking risks but does offer significant reasons for avoiding risks.

If employees are motivated to organize bargaining units, they will use their time, talent, and energy to force management to do their bidding. Of course, they could also use their time, talent, and energy to fulfill the organization's mission, support its values, and achieve its vision. To produce the latter result, executives must create an environment in which organizing a bargaining unit becomes unthinkable for employees. The real issue, then, is not how to motivate but how to *direct* and *manage* the motivation of managers, trustees, physicians, and employees.

3. *"Motivation never lasts."* In fact, behaviors do burn out and enthusiasm wanes when employees are driven exclusively by external rewards. However, employees will sustain performance when they internalize behavior and accept it as their own. Indeed, once employees have internalized a behavior, they will maintain it under the most difficult circumstances. By contrast, if external factors such as money or fear are used exclusively to provide motivation, performance will ebb and flow in direct relationship to the presence or absence of the reward or threat. For example, a primary care nurse who works in the emergency room simply because she

is paid a premium will probably never perform at the same level as a nurse who believes that the emergency room is the most exciting area of the hospital.

4. *"People need to be continually motivated."* All people are motivated 100 percent of the time. Motivation cannot be created; it can only be directed. The best way to direct motivation is to match the values and goals of the organization to the individual's values. When people see "the good" in their work, they perform at high levels because of the greater benefits to all. They feel a part of something bigger.

5. *"Staff motivation takes too much time."* Motivation may indeed take a great deal of time and money if the goal is to perform the organizational equivalent of changing the axis of the earth. For example, if the goal is to help the medical director behave more like an executive, it may take a long time to achieve that goal. Whether or not it is worth the time depends on how much that physician will help fulfill the organization's mission. However, working with key leaders to improve one small staff behavior a month is easy. Leaders think small, move fast, and celebrate often. When starting a new service, set small, achievable goals so staff can gain confidence in their new responsibilities. Even daily goals may be prudent in the beginning.

6. *"In the present health care environment, it takes longer to motivate employees."* Despite pressures from business, government, payers, and consumers, motivation takes no more time today than it did in the years before prospective payment. It is just that, in today's environment, motivating people to adapt to change seems to take longer because of the pace and volume of change. Health care executives are frightened and rush to reestablish control to give themselves a sense (illusion) of security. If we rush to reestablish control in the midst of chaos, people will seek safety. They will circle their wagons and dig their trenches.

7. *"The only real motives are fear and greed."* In reality, the only things that direct motivation are consistency of values and role clarity. A strong culture offers clearly understood roles, a bridge between past and present expectations, and support for taking risks and moving ahead to achieve the organization's vision. In a weak culture, however, employees are often confused about what manage-

ment expects and wants, and they fail to understand why the old way is no longer adequate. Fearing reprimand, they avoid innovation and risk taking. Thus, leaders motivate by matching what employees value with what the organization values.

8. *"Employees can't be treated the same way as managers."* The reality is that the more employees understand the organization's mission, accept its values, and share in the achievement of its vision, the deeper will be their commitment to the organization. If employees feel disenfranchised, they will stay around for their paychecks and may even modify their behavior if threatened with termination. But the data-processing manager, the accountant, and the quality assurance coordinator will perform at top levels only when they understand in what ways their work makes a difference to the organization. It must be impressed on the parking garage attendant that a friendly greeting to patrons is important to the hospital's reputation for high-quality service, and on the person who delivers food trays to patients how hot or cold food can affect their overall perception of care.

9. *"With some people, it's carrots; with others, it's sticks."* People can be motivated temporarily to carry out difficult or unattractive activities through a balance of rewards and threats. In an effective health care organization, however, carrots and sticks become unnecessary because people understand how they fit into the organization and contribute to its goals. Health care leaders must give meaningful recognition to the achievements of employees and minimize the threat of punishment. Self-managed employees create their own carrots and sticks.

Myths of mission and motivation shape and direct myths of management. If health care executives believe that a mission statement is little more than window dressing and that people are little more than interchangeable parts of a well-oiled machine, they will cling to outmoded concepts of executive behavior. They will view their role as managing material assets rather than human assets, and, while they may build bigger organizations, they will not make them more effective.

Health care leaders have one purpose: to build commitment to the organization's mission, values, and vision. But this requires that employees understand who they are, the purpose of their work, and how they can contribute to the success of the organization. Employees crave the locus of control found in a values-based mission as well as a vision they can accept and apply to their work lives. In this, the role of health care leadership is critical. If those in charge treat people like machines and continually look for new buttons to push, they will behave like machines and perform—but only until they fulfill a narrow assignment. If they have both responsibility and freedom, they will perform for the organization, not just for themselves.

Myths of Management

1. *"Top management doesn't have time to worry about people."* The reality is that just as Peter Drucker's symphony conductor worries about the score and having the right musicians, leaders invest 50 to 80 percent of their time creating an environment that will heighten the contribution of the work force. If executives are continually obsessed with buildings, financial reports, and legal briefs, employees will quickly get the message. It doesn't really make any difference what we do here, they may conclude. If managers want to worry about money and projects, we'll give them something new to worry about—we'll organize. If management won't talk to us as individuals, maybe it will talk to a bargaining unit. Executives who have no time to worry about people may be forced to take time when a collective bargaining unit is recognized or when people leave in large numbers. When employees feel exploited, they will not commit to the organization. But when they feel some ownership, anything that doesn't help the organization seems like a waste of time.

2. *"My role is to build an organization."* The reality is that an organization's greatest asset is not its strategic plan or balance sheet but its human capital. Thomas J. Watson, while president of IBM, made the following statement:

> I firmly believe that any organization, in order to survive and achieve success, must have a sound set of beliefs on which it premises all of its policies and actions.
>
> Next I believe that the most important single

factor in corporate success is faithful adherence to those beliefs.

And finally, I believe that if an organization is to meet the challenge of a changing world, it must be prepared to change everything about itself except those beliefs as it moves through corporate life.

In other words, the basic philosophy, spirit, and drive of an organization have far more to do with its relative achievements than do technological or economic resources, organizational structure, innovation, and timing. All these weigh heavily in success. But they are, I think, transcended by how strongly the people in the organization believe in its precepts and how faithfully they carry them out [1963, pp. 5–6].

3. *"Loyalty can't be created."* Leaders generate loyalty by being loyal. If you show care and concern for people, they will respond in the same way. Recently, a health care system closed down a hospital, moved employees twenty miles away to another hospital, and still increased commitment and job satisfaction in the work force. How? Because on day one, the CEO stood before his employees and said, "No one will get hurt. No one will lose his or her pension, and to the best of our ability, no one will leave here professionally damaged. However, we need to shut down this hospital and move most of you to a new hospital across town. Some of you won't go. Some of you may not want to go. We want to do this as fairly and compassionately as possible. So let's work together."

Following this meeting, the organization turned to its values-based mission to help employees understand the importance of closing the hospital. As a result, each employee could conclude, I'm contributing to the betterment of this community by working myself out of a job in this location. There is a good greater than my interests.

Leading Others by Managing Change

The leader's primary role is to build a strong culture by modeling the organization's mission, values, and vision. This sets the tone for interaction within the work force. The goal is to create an organization of self-managed people who understand their role in fulfilling the organization's values-based mission and achieving its vision. The effective health care leader communicates the purpose of the organization to every one of its members—from the chairperson of the board to the security guard and the physical therapist.

Frederick Brown, president of Christian Health Services (CHS) in St. Louis, understands the power of communication in building a strong corporate culture. Brown and his executives have developed a strong team by clarifying the values-based mission and vision of CHS. He has met with all staff within the system and explained the culture of CHS. To prove that he means what he says, he hands out his business card and tells staff to call him with their concerns. His card also has the mission of CHS printed on it. Frederick Brown is an excellent leader because he understands the importance of culture, teamwork, communication, and trust. He is CHS's best role model.

Consider an example. Does a mother, a father, two children, a house in the suburbs, and two cars add up to a family? Not necessarily, unless the members of one family are united by bonds of love and trust. Something similar is true of health care organizations. The mere fact that a hospital has a CEO, a board, a medical staff, and strategic and financial plans does not make it an effective hospital. Like strong and happy families, effective organizations have shared values, a "magical" quality, a spirit—a strong culture based on shared beliefs and common goals. Ideas emerge and the organization moves forward because of the underlying values that pervade and sustain everyone. Frederick Brown knows this formula.

It is often said that the best teams are not necessarily those with the best athletes; the best teams are those with the best coaches. Like the winning coach, the health care leader is pivotal in creating and building meaning for the work force. The following happens again and again: A leader leaves an organization, and another competent professional takes his place. No one knows why, but things are never quite the same again. "I don't know what's going on," moaned a hospital vice-president. "I'm doing everything my predecessor did, but I'm not getting the same results." What this executive failed to realize is that the first leader gave the organization something intangible: inspiration, esprit de corps, camaraderie, a sense of pride and joy that can never be replicated by simply adhering to policies and procedures.

For many health care executives, focusing their organizations on issues such as mission, values, and vision will not be easy. If you find that to be true of yourself, try to keep these concepts in mind:

Change is a process, not an event. It involves much more than creating a new business venture or delegating a pet project. When it comes to changing management styles, quick fixes never work. Such changes are far more complicated than installing a new software package or telephone system. Instead, you are trying to change people, many of whom have practiced the same behaviors for decades.

Change is a personal experience. Not everyone in the organization will respond to it in the same way. Nurses may embrace your efforts, while those in finance may ridicule it as "soft stuff." Be prepared to adapt your change program to individual needs and idiosyncrasies.

Change is experiential. The reality of change cannot be communicated through memos, slide presentations, videos, or brochures. Change will occur only when people experience the process and sense the excitement that comes from reshaping an organization. The more meaningful experiences people share, the more they will change their feelings and behavior.

Change must be expressed in practical, how-to terms. The key to successful change is helping members of the work force understand what change can mean for them. In what new ways will they perform their jobs? Will they feel differently about their co-workers? What problems will they attempt to solve? Leaders always clarify roles and expectations.

Keep the process simple. No matter how many workbooks are purchased, no matter how many seminars or lectures are sponsored, the final responsibility for change rests with the individual.

In the midst of the change process, it is not uncommon for health care executives to regress to past management styles. Given that reality, you should create a team of "organizational spotters," that is, trusted colleagues who understand the necessity of changing the organization. If your management style does begin to regress, these spotters can provide confidential feedback on how, when, and where the change process fell off the track. In addition, they can offer alternatives for dealing with the situation.

Following are some suggestions for introducing and executing a managed change process: First, start with a clear mission, a short list of core corporate values, and a well-defined vision. Second, let employees and staff members know that executives want to work with them in creating a strong corporate culture based on the organization's mission, values, and vision. They need to know that they are critical to the success of the undertaking. Third, explain that while building a more effective organization is the primary focus, change must also occur within the individual. Remind employees that they must all take a fresh look at their actions, values, and perceptions. Fourth, solicit feedback on your leadership style. Some typical questions might be: How is my behavior being received? How should I modify my behavior? What should I do differently, how should I do it, and why would a new approach be more successful? Fifth, prepare the management team for regression and backsliding. Remind your closest associates and subordinates that managed change is evolutionary and that a certain amount of regression and backsliding are inevitable.

Finally, suggest that members of the management team make themselves psychologically bulletproof. Ask them to remain objective and to take care not to personalize anything. Suggest that they respond to any backsliding on your part with, "I don't appreciate your behavior, but I'll do what you tell me to do because you're the boss."

In moving through the change process, remember that one person cannot alone produce change. A conductor produces no music without the orchestra; a football coach is not on the field with the players. All members of the team must be willing to change. Nevertheless, wanting change is almost never enough. Neither is a well-written action plan. Within the organization, four or five individuals may lack the values, skills, or knowledge to help the organization become more effective. Perhaps some of these individuals will be able to make the necessary adjustments, but others will inevitably leave. If the decision is that the orchestra will no longer play Sousa marches but progressive jazz, this will be bad news for the sousaphone player!

Building commitment to the organization's vision is the ultimate goal of the change process. Leaders understand the ten most important ways to build commitment during a managed change process:

1. Engagement: Involve all the people who will be affected by a program or system.
2. Create a "no-fault transfer" norm: Everyone loses when one loses.
3. Negotiate win-win solutions: Success is defined by how many individuals succeed.
4. Use goal clarity to focus each employee on his or her task: Create an organizational context (vision) for all tasks; this provides meaning and gives the employee purpose.
5. Emphasize the dynamics of change: There are no quick fixes; you must be flexible; bend don't break; change *will* continue to accelerate.
6. Focus on the human components of quality, achievement, and profitability.
7. Use data to promote commitment: Dx precedes Rx.
8. Adopt change strategies throughout the hospital and focus on systemic problems.
9. Create a positive vision: Look upon problems as challenges and opportunities and be proactive.
10. Nurture a sense of teamwork: Staffs with members who care for each other are more successful than those with members who are indifferent or hostile to one another.

Some employees, however, may simply refuse to change. In fact, they will do whatever they can to sabotage and discredit change efforts. For whatever reason—self-protection, tradition, security— they want no part of a new and different organization. You must therefore pose this question for every key player in the organization: How much are you willing to invest in the success of this enterprise? Staff members with low commitment to the organization must be either retrained or replaced with individuals who are willing to strengthen the culture.

Ask tough questions. To what extent is each person invested in the organization's success? What is gained by clinging to the past or the status quo? Realize that if staff lacks complete commitment

to the process, there may be problems bringing the organization
along.

Arthur Sturm, president of the Sturm Communications
Group in Chicago, has taken his company forward by managing
the change process and building commitment. A successful entrepreneur, Sturm knew that he had to build a new corporate culture
if his company were to continue to grow. His personal energy had
made the company a success. However, to accommodate market-
driven growth, he needed a team committed to his new vision of a
broad-based, customer-oriented company and he had to build additional strengths in his management team. He had to destroy the old
culture that was driven by the belief that Arthur Sturm, "our guru,"
would find a solution to any problem. Through a slow and sometimes frustrating managed change process and patience with those
staff members who needed constant reassurance, Sturm completely
rebuilt his culture by creating a team committed to his vision.

Chapter Three

Gaining
Organizational Commitment

To become a better leader, you must first understand a few basic principles of human motivation—specifically, you must understand what motivates people to work. Psychodynamic, developmental, biophysical, and behavioral theories are useful in explaining many kinds of human behavior. However, they are not the best models to explain leadership and organizational behavior. Let us turn instead to Maehr and Braskamp's *The Motivation Factor: A Theory of Personal Investment*. Their book looks at motivation from the standpoint of how people spend their time, talent, and energy. Consider your own behavior. How do *you* spend your time? When you get a series of phone calls, in what order do you return them? Of even more significance, whom do you call at noon or 5:00 P.M. because you know they probably will not be in their offices? In contrast, whom do you call right away?

We frequently exhibit conflicts between our words and our actions. In fact, the biggest problem that we have as health care professionals is that *we lie to ourselves*. For example:

- An executive claims he is caring, sensitive, and compassionate. But if he spends six months a year worrying about his hospital's budget and another six months defending it, where does the truth lie?

- Financial managers report their net operating margin to three decimal points but have no sense of their organization's core values. They pay lip service to care for the poor but offer only a 2 percent write-off as evidence of their concern. If these health care executives really wanted to care for the poor, wouldn't they invest more of their time, talent, and energy in doing so?
- In speeches and annual reports, executives may speak often and eloquently of the quality of care offered by their institutions. However, the nurses confide to colleagues, "We're pressured to make money; we're a profit center." Behavior and motivation are driven solely by the organization's desire to safeguard its economic position.

To know why people work, watch how they spend their time, talent, and energy. To know what they value most, take a look at task perseverance. People stay with tasks that are motivating but procrastinate when the task fails to "turn them on." If a manager takes only a week to write a proposal for a new marketing program but consistently submits her variance reports a month late, that provides a fairly clear notion of what makes her tick. Good intentions and well-meaning words are not behavior. Claiming to be motivated to do something serves no purpose if the person does not persevere at the behavior. What does it matter if an administrative assistant claims he is working hard but makes fifteen personal calls per day, fails to come in on time, takes long lunches, and consistently leaves early?

As a health care leader today, you must learn to focus on the frequency and duration of employee's behaviors if you want to determine what drives and motivates them. As an exercise, observe two or three managers or employees for two weeks. Watch what they do and how often they do it, as well as how long a given behavior lasts. Assessing what it would take to change their behavior will give you a fairly clear idea of the strength of their motivation—that is, where they are investing their time, talent, and energy.

Four Key Values

Ultimately, the motivation to invest personally in work lies in the relation of an employee's values to corporate values. According to *The Motivation Factor,* there are four values that shape personal investment: (1) recognition, (2) accomplishment, (3) power, and (4) affiliation. Recognition and accomplishment deal with how staff members relate to work, job, task, or activity, while power and affiliation pertain to people, relationships, friends, and colleagues.

Recognition. Some workers crave attention. They continually seek feedback on the quality of their work from their bosses and colleagues. To be seen as high-producing winners is all-important to them. They enjoy seeing their names in print, winning awards, and receiving public recognition at special events. For these workers, the emphasis is on external reinforcement of good work through verbal and written plaudits, awards, perks, supplemental benefits, and merit and salary increases.

Accomplishment. In their offices by 7:30 A.M., some employees race through project after project. They are eager to get involved in new ventures in the hope of achieving ever greater things. Anchored to their desks, these workers rarely take time out for lunch or routine conversation. In their professional life they emphasize productivity, doing the job right, and exploring new opportunities.

Power. Other staff members just want to win. They enjoy going head-to-head with the president of the medical staff, the chairperson of the city planning council, or anyone else. Instead of feeling intimidated by escalating competition from neighboring hospitals, they are exhilarated by it. Their professional life is driven by competition and conflict and the quest for power and position.

Affiliation. Finally, others want to create a family feeling among their staff members. They invest at least one-third of their day trying to build an atmosphere of trust and camaraderie among their employees. Birthdays, anniversaries, graduations, and births are celebrated with lunches and receptions. When an employee has a personal or family problem, they take time to talk it through with him and suggest solutions. Their professional life is driven by a desire to care for and respect their employees and to treat them as part of the hospital family.

Everyone is motivated by these four needs, but to varying degrees. Among executives, power tends to be the dominant value; however, the percentages of other values can shift as a result of circumstances. For example, the need for recognition might accelerate when a person feels threatened, and the value of accomplishment might jump dramatically during a budget crunch. But even if the values of recognition and accomplishment expand at times, they will always be subordinate to the dominant motivational value of power.

Some Typical Patterns

Are there typical values patterns for different types of professions? Looked at from the standpoint of *The Motivation Factor,* the typical health care professional is high in affiliation, medium high in power, and medium in recognition and accomplishment. A salesperson, in contrast, tends to be high in accomplishment, recognition, and power but low in affiliation. A successful health care leader is typically medium in power and recognition, and high in accomplishment and affiliation.

Emphasizing one value rather than another is not good or bad in itself. The problem begins when there is a conflict between the kinds of values that employees have and the kinds of values that the organization needs. For example, strategic plans often emphasize high recognition, accomplishment, and power values. But these plans would stand a greater chance for success if they were built on high accomplishment, medium power and affiliation, and medium-low recognition. The point is that leaders recognize that the value structures of the employees and the organization may differ. Leaders accept those differences and work to build strong cultures that align organizational values with employees' personal values.

When a personal value system fails to align with job expectations and the organization's core values, serious problems may result. For example, after thirty years in Catholic health care, a member of a religious order will have too many values in conflict if asked to run a for-profit subsidiary. In the same way, a hard-driving MBA just off the plane from Nashville will have little patience with extended dialogues on the need for compassionate care.

Matching personal with organizational values is the most critical challenge of leadership. The difficulty here, of course, is that each individual sees the world through his or her own eyes. A marketing vice-president with the dominant value of accomplishment has trouble seeing why her staff likes to adjourn a half hour early on Friday afternoons and go out for a drink, or why her secretary resents receiving a stack of written directives at 4:00 P.M. In the same way, a hospice director whose dominant value is affiliation may view her power-driven, numbers-focused vice-president of professional services as unfeeling. Or nurses who have given their lives to caring for patients and their families may have difficulty relating to physicians driven by power and accomplishment.

Does this mean that leaders should surround themselves with colleagues and subordinates who share the same dominant work values? No. If an affiliation-oriented human resources director hires staff who are exclusively driven by affiliation, the human resources function will probably suffer. People will spend so much time socializing with each other that nothing will get done. Although a group of highly affiliative nurses can usually work well together, a highly affiliative senior management group could run an institution into the ground in two years. In the same way, a heavy-hitting, power-oriented chief information officer might lock horns and do battle with a data-processing manager for whom power is an equally strong value. In such cases, one can only hope that a third party will emerge to coax the power-driven executives into opposite corners and refocus the combatants on their roles in achieving the organization's vision. Otherwise, the urge to dominate, compete, control, and win may come to obsess them.

Leaders surround themselves with diverse people. On an intuitive level, they understand dominant values and motivational drives and choose people who complement their style. Robert Fanning, president of Beverly Hospital in Beverly, Massachusetts, built an effective team from widely diverse, although exceptionally competent, staff members. Understanding the values of recognition, accomplishment, power, and affiliation helped Mr. Fanning to comprehend the dynamics of his team. His ability to focus such an intelligent and high-energy group demonstrates his leadership and explains his organization's success.

If a person views himself as a power-oriented executive who is more likely to persevere at a task for the sake of winning rather than out of relish for the task itself, that person should put together a team of people who rank high on the values of recognition, affiliation, and accomplishment. He should find people who can work hard and who will commit themselves to his vision and be loyal to the organization.

Keep in mind that power is not a negative. Leadership is power used positively. The power of leadership is defined not by what you say or believe, but by the people who are willing to stand behind you. If an executive declares, "We're going to move in this direction," and staff says, "You're nuts," that executive may have authority, but he is not a leader. Power only comes from his title—not his soul.

In the final analysis, leaders need to understand and manage all four values. Consider the analogy of the human body. To have a body that was all heart, muscle, brain or nervous system would be dysfunctional. A human being needs all these organs and systems. In the same way, an organization needs a balance of values: accomplishment (the head), affiliation (the heart), power (the muscular system), and recognition (the nervous system). Truly outstanding leaders, such as Robert Fanning, understand the interactive dynamics of these values and can balance them in such a way as to put the *right person* in the *right job* in the *right corporate culture.*

Let us therefore examine each of these values and see how they are expressed in terms of a corporate culture.

Values in the Environment

Many people invest a great deal of time and money to present themselves in certain ways. Ambience and environment offer clues to a leader's dominant values and expectations of others.

Recognition. Is the office a shrine filled with plaques and autographed photos taken with political and other celebrities? This executive craves attention, and you can motivate her by recognizing and praising her performance.

Accomplishment. Is this an office that features halogen lights, a FAX machine, an electronic dictionary, worksheets, and a desk PC? Offer this executive well-edited data and information at a brisk pace. Time is this leader's currency.

Power. Is this office dominated by an enormous, pristine mahogany desk, credenza, and conference table? Expect power-driven responses. A bookshelf contains a few select awards and national best-sellers on executive leadership. This person is a competitor, someone who wants to win and who enjoys gaining authority and control over others. Be prepared for some good-natured verbal jousting.

Affiliation. Is this a plain but immaculate office decorated in soft, muted tones? A crucifix and other religious mementos may be displayed prominently. This leader rises from his desk to greet you and asks how you are feeling. In working with this person, expect him to place emphasis on building a team and to go out of his way to help others on the team.

Values in Evaluation

Performance evaluations show clearly the dominant work values of the evaluator. Many times the evaluation process shows more about the evaluator than the one being evaluated.

Recognition. The executive motivated by recognition wants to believe that an employee's successful performance is a direct result of the executive's strong leadership. His evaluation of an employee might sound like this: *"I'm* really concerned about how you feel about this evaluation and your work here at Health, Inc. *I'd* like to spend some time discussing how *I* helped increase your effectiveness this year and how *I* can help you even more in the year to come. *I've* noticed that you've really thrived since you transferred into *my* division a year ago. *I* think you'll agree that *I've* really done a great job in developing some of your outstanding skills and talents. *I'm* really pleased you were able to mesh with *me* and produce such dramatic results for *my* hospital. You've really grown under *my* leadership."

Power. The power-oriented executive tends to challenge an employee's behavior and often suggests that the employee emulate her style. An evaluation typically goes like this: "The way you handled those industrial clinic joint ventures showed some inconsistencies in judgment. If you look back at how the gallstone lithotripter was handled, you'll get a better idea of where you could have gained an edge. You could have questioned harder and received more concessions. We play hardball here, and next year you need to stiffen your spine and tough out better negotiations. You've got the right talent and education. But you need to push harder, because next year is going to be even tougher than this year. You did all right this year, but we're in this game to win over the long haul." "There are only Ws (winners) and Ls (losers)—if you behave like an L, you're history!"

Affiliation. The affiliation-oriented executive openly shares information and shows care and concern for the employee's welfare. He would begin an evaluation this way: "How are you feeling today? Well, it looks like it's time for your evaluation again. I hope this is a good day for you. Before we sit down and talk, why don't you take some time and review the evaluation form I've completed? We'll probably need quite a bit of time to discuss this, so why don't you clear your calendar for the rest of the day? I don't think there's anything in here that's going to upset you, but I know this is really important to you, and I want this to be a positive experience. Now, if it's not helpful, I want you to please tell me about it. You know you can talk to me. I think you know how I feel about your being with us and how much you've helped us all."

Accomplishment. The executive who is accomplishment-oriented sees success as a matter of meeting corporate objectives. His fast-moving, staccato evaluations often leave employees breathless: "OK, you met your department's first five strategic objectives, but you're still working on those last two. Let's look at next year. I think we've got some fairly strong criteria. I've got to tell you, you've got a bunch of people over there, but you don't have a team, you know what I mean? You've got some real all-stars, but I don't see them working together. You know what I'm saying? Now, I want to see real force there next year. Let's get all that energy moving in one direction. It's not there yet. When will it happen?

Values in Decision Making

Executives with certain value profiles also have unique ways of making decisions.

Power. The power-oriented executive may create a facade of participation, involvement, and consensus, but the decision she wants has already been made. Her skill is in getting others to agree to and buy into that decision and in taking control of implementation. When she makes a decision, she sticks with it. To do otherwise is to "lose!"

Recognition. The recognition-oriented executive takes credit for decisions. He gives special emphasis to how he personally resolved conflicts, involved others, and gathered information during the arduous decision-making process. According to his account, there would have been no decision if it were not for his outstanding skills in negotiation, problem solving, and consensus building. All he craves is recognition as the team's savior and spiritual guide. "See what I did for you. Yet again, I showed you how important I am."

Affiliation. The affiliation-dominated executive often has problems making decisions. He goes out of his way to ensure that everyone contributes to and feels good about a decision. Because he feels compelled to seek continual feedback from others, he hesitates to announce a final decision. If a decision is made quickly, he worries that he may not have gotten everyone's input. In the worst case, he will sacrifice a decision. If a power-oriented colleague declares, "I don't want to do that. I've got a better idea," he may respond, "OK, that sounds like a good idea."

Accomplishment. The accomplishment-oriented executive wants data and action—and he wants it now. He sweeps people into action by urging them to clear their calendars so that they can get together and hammer out a plan. He quickly mobilizes all the resources—from outside consultants to off-site retreat locations—that will be needed to get the job done. Echoing themes of innovation, challenge, and opportunity, he decides quickly and has little patience for people who do not understand the need to move ahead rapidly.

Chapter Four

Ensuring
Motivated Employees

Every corporation has three parts: the personalities of the employees hired to do a job, the characteristics of the job that the employees were hired to do, and the culture of the organization in which the employees perform their jobs.

Whether they came to your health care organization as nurses, laboratory technicians, or vice-presidents, people bring with them a history of personal experience and technical knowledge. The jobs that they perform give them an opportunity to build on their experience and expand their skills while the corporate culture gives purpose and pride to them. Leaders must constantly try to fit the right person into the right job within a meaningful culture. When this happens, employees become self-managed, motivated, and productive.

Matching Personal and Corporate Values

No employee is a tabula rasa. When you hire people, you hire their whole history—experiences, skills, and knowledge. A strong leader understands that running an effective organization starts with hiring the right person. The next step is to put this skilled and motivated person into a job where her values and technical skills can flourish. Then the leader continues to build an organizational culture that allows the person to grow in direct proportion to the organization's success. When the person, job, and organization are moving in the same direction toward a common goal, the organization is effective. But if one element is out of alignment, there is likely to be trouble. A talented and gifted nurse with a rich history of caring can easily get a job in the corporate nursing department of a for-profit multihospital system. Once there, she may find that she enjoys her work but that she dislikes the system. Her alternatives are to do her job while psychologically disengaging herself from the system, adapt to the new value system, or leave.

The situation for nurses is especially poignant. In years past, hospitals were seen as places where patients received care and got well. Today, they are sometimes viewed as costly production lines where very sick people are "fixed" and sent home. Caring clinicians are being forced to embrace industrial engineering productivity models. Many nurses have grown disenchanted because the culture of caring has disappeared from so many hospitals. Whereas a nurse may once have reported to the director of nursing, she now reports to a product-line manager whose goal is to make sure that services contribute to the hospital's business objectives. She may feel comfortable and fulfilled when doing traditional nursing but anxious and resentful when managing a profit center or engaging in cost control and charge capture.

Nurses are facing a conflict between their personal values (why did I enter this profession?), their backgrounds, and technical skills, as well as a clash between today's economically driven health care environment and their own expectations. A person who served the nursing profession for twenty years now finds herself being told, however subtly, that her behavior is somehow wrong or inadequate. If the organization is clumsy about communicating the reasons for necessary changes, it will be increasingly difficult for that nurse to function—no matter how much she likes giving patient care.

Health care executives face a similar dilemma. Health care executives over forty years of age probably came out of a MHA program in the early 1970s with a heavy dose of history and public health. Their role was to work with trustees on fund development and new building projects and to give physicians whatever they requested. The current numbers-focused, MBA mentality runs counter to their experience and education. In order to cope, a health care executive probably depends on one of three strategies:

1. *Denial:* "I don't know how to cope with this, but I really don't think the situation is as serious as most people make out. The government will probably tire of this in a few years and we'll go back to the old system."
   Result: Loss of job or early retirement.
2. *Dependency:* "I don't have the psychological resources to cope with this. I wasn't trained as a cost accountant. I'm going to do what I've always done best and leave this cost stuff to the financial guys."
   Result: Abrogation of significant power to the CFO and possible loss of job.
4. *Leadership:* "Something's happened but we're going to survive this no matter what it does to other hospitals. We're going to pool our resources and find out what it means for us."
   Result: Inspired people with a new culture that confronts the demands of PPS and seeks solutions appropriate to the organization. There is a good chance that this executive will thrive regardless of the velocity or volume of change because he has created a team spirit among the work force that enables it to achieve his vision.

Providing Resources

The ability of an organization to grapple with change depends on the amount of meaningful involvement opportunities it creates for employees. If it can help employees see that change is necessary and will produce specific benefits, the organization will be able to move forward. As a leader, it is your role to help all employees deal with change. When the next change is considered, look at who will be most threatened by change and try to understand their dynamics and background. If their values and history conflict with new expectations, work with them. Assure them that while their beliefs and values are still valid, they must now develop new behaviors, such as better record keeping and charge capture to control cost and enhance profitability. Explain how their behavior will help the organization move forward and become more effective. Most importantly, support them with staff development that ensures that they have the skills to perform their new tasks.

Leaders must provide the resources to help people change. For example, one problem is that there is no academic curriculum for change management. Clinical supervisors often end up performing more clinical than actual supervisory functions because that is what they know how to do. They are unable to delegate authority or control or manage conflict because they never learned how. Managing change must be learned, and this means acquiring new skills and practicing them. Leaders are successful in moving organizations in new directions—product-line management, sales and marketing, managed care—because they offer programs that support and inspire their employees.

Does this mean that everyone can learn how to work in a new organization and environment? No, some employees will not make it. Although every worker deserves an opportunity, change is more difficult for some people than for others. Updating old skills and building new ones are relatively easy, but it is almost impossible to change people who have rigid values. Staff who lead verbal assaults with statements such as, "In my last job, we didn't do it that way," "We've never done it this way before," and "It won't work; we tried it ten years ago," may never come around to the new way of doing things. Leaders must wish them the best but remove them compassionately because they don't fit.

In the same way, a skilled and valued CFO with an authoritarian personality will probably no longer fit in an organization that is evolving from a vertical, command/control structure to an information-based, fast-acting one. If the CFO pays lip service to independence and faster response times but still sends combative memos to staff in member hospitals, he is dysfunctional. No amount of counseling, education, or discussion will reduce the impact that his past training, personal values, and history have on his behavior. He must be replaced.

In other cases managers' technical skills might be excellent, but their values cause them to be dysfunctional and disruptive. A hard-nosed MBA with a for-profit bent may seem to be everything you want in a new business director, but her experiences may run counter to the organization's culture of shared responsibility. As a result, she may well become frustrated with the organization, making demands that are impossible to fulfill.

Like everything else, people, jobs, and organizations change. The environment exerts unending and irregular pressures on organizations. In response they must redesign their cultures and "retool" their workers. New cultures and structures call for new kinds of people. Today's health care leaders must figure out what the organization needs and help people change to meet the future. In the same way, leaders must evaluate workers in two ways: what they are now and what they must become if they are to contribute to the organization in the years ahead.

Finally, leaders must think about what their organizations will become and communicate this vision in all things—especially in the use of human capital. A leader knows that because health care is a service business, the corporation's greatest assets are not on the balance sheet—they are walking the halls. Health care leaders are rethinking who they are, what business they are in, and whether they have the right team. And, once they have defined their business and culture, they must clarify the roles of each team member and find the best people to execute these roles. Remember: leaders inspire.

The leader's most elemental task is to balance what the organization expects of its employees with the employees' capacity to meet those expectations. Employees who are matched carefully to a job will rarely quit or become troublemakers, because they feel committed and bonded to the organization. If an organization has a reputation as a "revolving door," its executives must question their leadership ability. What happens between the time new employees walk into their new offices and the day they return their ID badges to security? The events between these two points define the executive's ability to lead.

Unfortunately, in approaching recruitment, the ineffective health care executive uses the warm-body approach—if the applicants are breathing and have the right credentials, they are hired. However, there is a step that must be taken before employees are hired. That step is to formulate the organization's purpose (values and mission) and set its direction (vision). *Then* the best and the brightest people are found to achieve the vision. Trustees sometimes hire heavy-hitter CEOs from larger, more prosperous institutions only to fire them for bringing the organization "too far too fast" and "stepping on toes." In the same way, senior executives bring in superstars with skills and talent but no sense of team play. The best and the brightest are defined by their ability to maintain harmony, manage diversity, and coordinate effort in a particular culture. Leaders explore how the concepts of person, job, and organization apply to their own situation. In doing so, they resist such hasty conclusions as "we need twenty-five new nurses" or "we've got to get a marketing vice-president from industry." When addressing these issues, they ask the following kinds of questions: Is it a person, a job, or the organization that needs changing? What should the organization become? Do existing jobs match our mission, values, and vision? Do we have the right people to perform these jobs? If not, can these individuals be trained or coached, or should they be dismissed compassionately and replaced with others who fit the organization better?

Job Satisfaction and Commitment

Job satisfaction is the intangible result of a strong match between the person, the job, and the organization. Job satisfaction measures how happy employees are with their jobs, pay, co-workers, and supervisors. Commitment, however, is a measure of employee loyalty, pride, and ownership. Staff will be satisfied and committed when their jobs provide them with the opportunity to be self-managed and empower them to achieve the organization's vision.

To the surprise of many, there is a special relationship between compensation and job satisfaction. When staff are neither loyal or satisfied, they need to be paid more just to do the job.

Executives spend thousands of dollars on compensation studies when they should focus on the match between an employee's expectations and a job's opportunities. For example, if a nurse's personal need to care for patients matches the experiences available from working in an oncology unit, she will enjoy high job satisfaction, take pride in her work, and accept reasonable pay rates. But if a nurse is rotated through various units with no attention to how her needs match those of the unit, she will probably feel used and demand a pay differential. The message is clear: People must feel needed, respected, and competent. If the inherent aspects of the job do not provide these elements, then the paycheck must or people will leave! People work for *both* financial income and psychic income. Psychic income results from the combination of commitment and job satisfaction. The less psychic income that employees receive, the more financial income they will demand. Leaders are generous with both but emphasize psychic income.

Even in the executive ranks, psychic rewards are highly important. When a senior executive feels anxious about her work or undervalued as a person, financial compensation becomes an almost seductive lure. She will continue to seek greater compensation or perks inside the organization or she will look outside for a more lucrative opportunity. The absence of intrinsic rewards coupled with chronic anxiety about performance will cause her to demand higher and higher pay.

Effective leaders are defined more by the commitment they engender in their followers than by the satisfaction they derive from their jobs. A director of dietary services may be satisfied with her job, but feel no commitment to the organization. She would have few reservations about going to a competitor to perform the same duties for a relatively modest increase in pay or for some other reward. Many "climate" surveys of hospitals with high turnover rates leave executives baffled because employees report that they are satisfied with their jobs. What these surveys fail to ask is a critical follow-up question: Are you committed to the success of this organization? Commitment is the number one by-product of effective leadership, and commitment is characterized by loyalty and pride.

Job satisfaction is typically measured by questions such as, Is there a match between your skills and experience? What does this job give you an opportunity to do? Do you like your boss? Is your compensation fair? Organizational commitment, in contrast, is measured by questions such as, What would cause you to leave this organization? Do you understand this organization's purpose and beliefs? Are you proud of this organization?

Employee groups that exhibit high levels of satisfaction but low levels of commitment place the organization at risk. People in these groups tend to retreat into small enclaves for support. They reinforce one another with comments such as, "Just do your job." "We don't know what they're doing over there, but we know our job." "Let's just do our work and go home." "A day's work for a day's pay."

Mind Stretcher

Consider your own level of job satisfaction and organizational commitment by answering yes or no to the following questions taken from MetriTech's *Healthcare Organizational Assessment Survey* (pp. 6–7). The Healthcare Organizational Assessment Survey (Larry A. Braskamp, Ph.D., and Martin L. Maehr, Ph.D.) is copyright © 1986 by MetriTech, Inc., 111 North Market Street, Champaign, IL. (217) 398-4868. Reproduced by permission.

Job Satisfaction

- My co-workers and I work well together.
- I feel I get sufficient pay for the work I do.
- I like what I'm doing here, so I don't think of doing anything else.
- I get rewarded in a fair way for the work I do.
- I like my chances of doing work here so I can get ahead.
- I'm satisfied with the opportunities I have to direct people in my work.
- I get along with my supervisor.
- I like the people I work with.
- I like the work I do.
- I have good job security.

Organizational Commitment

- I have a sense of loyalty to this organization.
- I identify with this organization.
- I think about the future of this organization.
- I regret that I chose to work with this organization.
- I like to work here because I want the organization to succeed.
- I feel that I share in the success and failure of this organization.

- I feel I have a sense of ownership in this organization.
- It would take a great deal for me to move to another organization.
- I take pride in being part of this organization.

Employees may like their job and co-workers but still feel no sense of identification with or loyalty to the organization. Those in the executive ranks may be in a slightly different situation. Traumatized by unrelentless change, they become obsessed by the details of their jobs and ignore the broader purposes of the organization. Continually looking ahead to the next meeting, financial statement, board agenda, or medical staff report, they manage their way through twelve-hour days. Because they have no idea of how their job fits the organization's purpose, their only recourse is to work harder, longer, and faster and become even busier. Such managers approach their job like a student cramming for finals: I just need to get a passing grade and move on. No commitment, no passion, no leadership!

When people leave an organization or begin to look for new jobs, it is usually because they experience low psychic and financial income. Comments made to friends and colleagues are telling:

Growth: "There's no opportunity for me to advance here. I'm going to look for another job."

Satisfaction: "If I stay here, they're going to have to pay me more, because I'm not happy with my job and I want more money."

Productivity: "I'm not productive here. I'm going to look for a job that values my contributions."

Frustration: "There's no relief in sight. Things aren't going to get better."

Priorities: "The organization needs skills I don't have, and I don't want to take the time, energy, and dollars to develop those skills."

Philosophy: "I don't like the way health care is going: I don't want to be part of it. I just want out."

Executives with few leadership skills will probably answer the following questions in quite different ways:

- What are my beliefs and values?
- What can I achieve as an executive and where can I do it?
- What am I really worth—as a person and as a professional?
- What are my most significant skills and talents?
- Does this job give me the opportunity to function with my strengths at least 80 percent of the time?

Although some executives continually seek new opportunities, others will try to mold an organization to fit their personalities and values. It is not uncommon to hear about the bright, aggressive, highly verbal CEO who turns a small community hospital into an entrepreneurial machine. Instead of leaving to become a superstar in a large organization, this leader makes the organization so vigorous and forward looking that he is never bored. He creates the conditions (defines the culture and builds the team) that make him more satisfied and committed.

Without commitment, an organization has nothing. High satisfaction without commitment will produce little more than a group of people who, when satisfiers weaken, may walk away and never take the time to wave goodbye. When staff are committed to an organization, however, there is unlimited potential for growth. The truly valuable manager is one who can say, "I believe in this place; the only way I would leave here is if the leadership changed." She may not be completely satisfied with her job, but she knows in which direction things are headed. She will invest her time, talent, and energy to help create a more effective organization because her deep belief in the leader's vision takes priority over superficial satisfiers.

Job satisfaction and commitment measures can also be used to anticipate and predict behavior. If employees have low organizational commitment, they may be candidates for union-organizing activities. And if employees have high job satisfaction and low commitment, the probability of union activity is especially strong because employees will want to protect their jobs. People with high commitment may not be satisfied with their jobs, but they love the organization and will put in time to make it more effective. Those with high satisfaction and low commitment are more likely to complain: "Why are we having all of these meetings? I have work to do.

I need to pay attention to my job, so stop bugging me with this mission stuff; it has nothing to do with me."

To build a more effective organization, a leader needs to produce high job satisfaction and high commitment. Keeping workers happy is not the answer, and, in many cases the existence of such workers may actually indicate an unwillingness to go the distance for the organization. If an executive is satisfied with his job but lacks commitment to the organization, he will eventually move elsewhere. Or if an executive without a solid values-based mission and supporting vision remains with an organization, he could someday be among the corps of shell-shocked executives who cry out, "How can you treat me like this? I've given my life to this organization. Doesn't that mean anything?"

Strengthening Your Culture

What makes a strong culture? Service awards? Holiday parties? Monthly staff and management meetings? A calendar of staff birthdays hung in the coffee room? Unfortunately, none of these things—alone or in combination—will create a strong culture. A salad bar in the cafeteria, a better parking spot, and an office with a view are the visual artifacts of an organization's climate—the things that can be seen. A culture, however, is based on beliefs. A strong culture exists when the following conditions are present:

- The organization has a clear sense of direction.
- Employees know what is expected of them.
- Employees embody the important values of the organization.

If a strong culture exists, employees will answer yes to three questions: Do I understand the mission, vision, and values of this organization? Do I share these values? Do I demonstrate them in my work?

In recent years, the cultures of health care organizations have been under almost continual attack. Executives thought they understood what hospitals did and why they existed. But what happens when the 200-bed hospital that stood at the corner for eighty years is forced to close and the other hospital in town finds it necessary to open a clinic in the mall? Executives in their late forties and fifties have been known to say, "I don't know what hospitals are anymore. I spent several years of my life getting an education and over twenty years in management, and I don't know where we're going or what we believe in."

Given their confusion about health care, hospitals, and their professional roles, it is no wonder that executives find it difficult to build a strong culture where everyone shares the same values. The problem is that all culture must start at the top—not in human resources and not with a service management program. A leader's most critical role is to define the culture, communicate the culture, and reward people who move the organization forward in the context of that culture. *A strong culture can never develop unless a leader first envisions it, articulates it, and lives it.*

What happens if the CEO abrogates this responsibility? Most likely, a mosaic of subcultures will emerge. No one can live outside a values context, which means that no one can live without a culture. If the CEO fails to define and promote a clear corporate culture, employees will often create conflicting subcultures. Confused by upper management talk about "a decentralized, polycorporate environment," finance may create a subculture devoted to controlling debt and watching over cash flow, the cash, budget, and accounts receivable. Other professionals and disciplines that are in the process of developing new identities, such as nursing, pharmacy, and physical therapy, will also create subcultures to define their context—the belief system that underpins their behavior.

An effective organization can and should have many diverse personalities, but only one corporate culture. In a strong culture, you can put people who are in clinical areas, support, or fund development in the same room and they will continue to talk care, support, and fund development—but in the context of the organization's mission, vision, and values. In ineffective organizations, diverse subcultures are less benign. If the vision is to create a responsive, information-based organization and the CFO exercises neurotic control over cash, debt, and capital, problems will arise. If an executive wants to build a diversified business group to cover losses in acute care units and the medical staff resists, there will be other kinds of problems. Dynamic tension is healthy for an organization as long as the members respond in unison, How does this help our purpose? Is this what we're working for?

In describing strong cultures, people often speak of vitality, exuberance, soul, energy, heart, magic, life. In short, strong cultures have *spirit*. They possess a dynamic energy even though their employees are relaxed, open, and friendly. Employees understand the big picture and do everything they can to help each other and the people they serve. Successful teams are not those with the greatest skill but those with the best spirit. If one team has 100 players who are confused, apathetic, and unfocused and the other team has 10 players who display a "magical" quality about winning, which team has the odds? It is never size—it is always spirit.

The hallmark of an effective organization is a focused, satisfied, and committed work force. If employees, physicians, and trustees are satisfied and committed, they will not only be productive but will thrive on change. Unfortunately, many executives introduce change with no understanding of corporate values and what motivates employees. When resistance mounts, they wail, "My staff is organizing. They don't understand. Why are they fighting me on this? I just spent $100,000 on a strategic plan and they won't implement it." If an executive pushes through a plan and ignores issues of values, satisfaction, commitment, and culture, he will likely double or triple the plan's original costs in turnover, reduced productivity, and internal strife and still never be able to implement the plan. Leaders realize that it is easy to formulate ideas and plans—success is found in implementation, not design.

CEOs who are hired into organizations with unfamiliar cultures have two choices: Adapt to the current culture and put a distinctive trademark on it or create a new culture. Some CEOs make the transition, but others crash and burn within ninety days, usually over a culture-related, values-based issue. The CEO who was once viewed by the board as the hope for the future quickly becomes the maniac who went out of control. The aggressive, entrepreneurial problem solver who was hired to catapult the organization into the twenty-first century is berated for "moving us too far too fast." CEOs are much more likely to lose their jobs because of a "personality conflict" than lack of competence.

Since behavior is driven by values, leaders should take time out once a year to do a total assessment of person, job, and organization to see how the values function and fit. They must be willing to ask some hard questions: How strong is the organization's culture? Do various subcultures have a negative impact? Are employees divisive or are they willing to sound the organization's battle cry? Where are values strong and where are they weak? Can the mission be achieved? Are the *right people* in the *right jobs* doing the *right things*? Does the organization have a soul? If yes, is it headed for heaven or hell?

PART TWO

Creating
a More Effective
Organization

Chapter Five

Identifying Needs
and Initiating Changes:
A Three-Phase Process

The goal of executive leadership is to create health care organizations with strong cultures. Understanding the relationship between a strong corporate culture and leadership requires an analysis of tangible and intangible input factors and output factors.

Consider Jeffrey Norman at Fitzgerald Mercy Hospital in Darby, Pennsylvania. It may not be immediately obvious that, as a young CEO, he has created an almost perfect balance between the tangible and intangible elements of his organization. However, if you followed him around for a while, you would learn that his passion for productivity and accountability is framed by an optimistic belief in the potential of people. He understands very clearly that effective organizations must take into account all the elements listed in Figure 1. Jeffrey Norman is a leader.

Most leaders want their employees to make a strong commitment to the organization. When this occurs, the organization will have a strong culture, and employees will exhibit job satisfaction, pride, and high morale. Therefore, if a leader creates a strong culture, he will have followers—highly committed people who are proud to work for him and the organization.

A leader's employees will display the sense of respect, trust, and well-being that results from the unique form of energy created

Figure 1. Elements of an Effective Organization.

	Tangibles	Intangibles
Input	Strategy Cash People Policy/Procedures Plant Information Systems Communication Systems	Culture Mission Values Vision Inspiration Leadership Style Motivation/Recognition
Output	Profit Market Share New Products Grow Diversify Productivity Quality	Commitment Morale Job Satisfaction Team Spirit Pride/Joy Trust Quality

by team spirit. They believe in their leader, and, without saying so directly, they acknowledge his ability to inspire the organization.

To assess her leadership ability, a leader must turn to her followers and ask these questions:

- Do you share the organization's beliefs?
- Do you like working here?
- Will you stay?
- Do people get along here?
- Do you feel proud of your work?
- Are you happy about working here?
- Is trust prevalent throughout the organization?

If most of the work force answers yes to these questions, this means that they are followers who have committed themselves to the vision of the organization. It would be a different conclusion if the work force answers the questions with "I don't know and I don't care."

Unfortunately, many health care organizations do not measure their success on the basis of intangible factors such as culture, morale, or commitment. Instead, they measure success on the basis of financially oriented, tangible variables such as profit, increased market share, and productivity.

The reality is that an organization may perform successfully in many of these areas but still lack leadership. An even deeper reality is that organizations that lose control of, minimize, or ignore the intangible factors will suffer in the tangible output sector. If the culture is weak and people feel no pride in their work and no commitment to the organization, then market share, profit, and productivity are at great risk. The situation is like a snake eating its own tail. It believes it is satisfying its appetite, until it bites its head.

Achieving Effectiveness

The three-phase process for creating a more effective organization—assessment, analysis, and action—begins with a thorough examination of the intangible elements that characterize such an organization. In medicine, treatment without diagnosis is malpractice. The same principle holds true for health care organizations. Unless data are first gathered about the organization, a diagnosis and a practical, workable course of treatment can never be developed. Just as a physician examines and talks with the patient, so a leader must scrutinize and interact with every component of the organization.

Central to this process are several issues: What is really happening to this organization? How are people being affected by the increasing pressure in health care to do more with less? Most importantly, what is the leader's personal style of leadership? Is it helping or hindering the organization in achieving its mission, fulfilling its values, and moving toward its vision?

Assessment. Although the word *assessment* may awaken painful memories of third-grade multiplication tests, or grades hidden from parents, organizational assessment is a direct, benign, and clear-cut process. Reduced to its simplest terms, organizational assessment involves two steps: The organization's behavior must first be translated into numbers, and it must then be established that the numbers are meaningful to the organization.

Essential to the assessment process is a leader's candid look at his own management style. In performing this self-appraisal, he must confront such basic issues as how he expresses his feelings and beliefs, communicates his vision, recognizes and rewards high performers, disciplines with compassion, and celebrates team accomplishments. Caution is necessary here. In digging beneath the surface, leaders may uncover troubling truths about how they perceive others. They should consider these questions:

- Do people in the organization really enjoy the process of working? What is the leader's role in facilitating satisfaction in the work place?
- To what extent does the leader operate with varying perceptions and expectations of the professional, management, technical, clerical, and support staff? How do these perceptions and expectations shape the behavior of the work force?
- What are the typical ways in which the leader refers to workers in conversations with colleagues, senior management, physicians, and trustees? What do these labels indicate about his attitudes, beliefs, and values?
- Are workers viewed simply as necessary evils or as cogs in the organizational machine? If not, how is their status as partners in fulfilling the organization's mission reinforced?
- How much credit is the work force given for organizational excellence? In the leader's role as orchestra conductor, how much acknowledgment do the musicians get as the primary reason for the organization's success?
- What specific actions have been taken in the last week, the last month, and the last year to show workers that they are valued? What have been the results of these efforts?

Analysis. Analysis requires both evaluation and judgment. Consider this example: Following an annual physical, a physician tells the patient that his cholesterol level is 340. The number is nothing more than the quantification of a condition at that moment in time. It is when the physician says "You know, this is quite serious" that she engages in evaluation. She is explaining that the number represents a negative or harmful situation. In assessment, behavior is frozen in time and then quantified. In the analysis phase, the raw data are evaluated, and a determination is made whether or not the data signify that the behavior is acceptable. Analysis is needed to interpret what those numbers mean in terms of the corporate culture. It is during the analysis phase that the following questions are asked and answered:

1. Why does our organization exist? (mission)
2. What do we believe in? (values)
3. Where are we headed? (vision)
4. Does everyone answer these questions in the same way? (strength of culture)

These are the four toughest questions that leaders must ask.

Action. It is during the action phase that leaders develop and implement the program for change. They identify and analyze barriers to achieving the vision and list the essential change elements, which are the positive alternative to behaviors that are blocking progress. They originate in key bottlenecks which, when changed, have dramatic effects. These change elements form a bridge between the organization's present and its future. The intangibles of mission, vision, and values address three issues: Why do we exist? What do we believe in? Where are we headed? What are the barriers or obstacles that we must eliminate, reduce, or accept? Essential change elements complete the statement: "In order to move forward, we must. . . ." Whether they involve hard assets or intangibles such as trust and cooperation, essential change elements redirect energy from barriers toward action.

Insight into the barriers to change and identification of the essential change elements create the road map for action, but, as the Nike commercial says, "Now, just do it!"

Assessment: Define Your Target

Assessing an organization involves measuring its intangible aspects (Figure 1). Assessment is the process whereby behaviors are converted into measurable, quantifiable statements. These raw data become the basis for analysis, judgment, and action plans. The difficult aspects of assessment are ensuring that whatever you decide to measure is in fact what you are measuring, that the results are valid and reliable for your organization, and that the data allow you to compare your organization against some norm. These conditions must exist before informed interpretations of the data can be made.

Shooting from the Hip. Health care executives sometimes approach organizational assessment as though it were a gunfight at high noon. Instead of addressing the factors that can result in victory or defeat, they come out with guns blazing and, in classic shoot-from-the-hip style, look for the most convenient or obvious target. As a result, many health care executives never take their finger off the trigger long enough to understand their organization's most troublesome intangible weaknesses or its deepest reservoirs of intangible strengths. Such lack of focus costs time, money, and effort. Recall the medical model. Treatment without diagnosis is malpractice. In the same way, in the executive ranks, data about the intangibles, converted by analysis into information, must drive every change program. If you don't measure, you can't manage!

"One Size Fits All." Someday we may live in a world where organizational development programs will be like pantyhose and stretch underwear: One size fits all. Unfortunately, like the less-than-perfect individuals who try to fit themselves into these miracles of Seventh Avenue, health care employees often feel squashed and uncomfortable when forced to undertake generic change programs. To address a complex intangible problem with a one-size-fits-all tangible solution is *always* a waste of time and money.

The matter of guest relations provides an example. Convinced that Marriott and Disneyland held the magic elixir to cure health care's ills, self-styled guest relations experts proceeded to wrap every wounded hospital with the same bandage. All too often, employees reacted with anger and resentment: "My mother taught me how to smile." "I don't need a script to do my job." "This isn't a hotel." The only truly effective patient satisfaction programs were those that were designed, pilot tested, and evaluated by the health care professionals who would use them. In these cases, the employees pinpointed the real problems, generated support from the lowest levels of the organization, and then concluded, We need a tiny refinement in this area and a major overhaul here. They owned the program—they were committed. All the leader did was inspire them to think about improving service.

This is not to say that there is no value in prefabricated programs. Workbooks—now frequently backed by computer software—can be helpful if managers use them to generate basic awareness, create insights, or remedy specific problems. There is no reason to develop a program if one with a good track record of success already exists. But permanent change only happens when the work is tailored to an organization's culture. Successful change comes from commitment and commitment comes from ownership.

Smoking causes 390,000 deaths a year, and morbid obesity is a risk factor for stroke, heart attacks, and diabetes. Does this mean that everyone who tries to quit smoking should go through hypnosis, biofeedback, acupuncture, massage therapy, or any number of other programs popular at the moment? The answer is no. Different techniques and strategies work for different people. Again, the upwardly mobile young accountant who successfully lost weight by means of a modified fast and liquid protein supplements may have a personality, education, and socioeconomic background that contributed to her success. The same program might not work for a hospital cafeteria worker whose identity revolves around cooking glorious meals for her family.

The analogy also applies to organizations. The 325-bed hospital in an upscale suburb wins over its employees with a sophisticated health promotion program that includes personal diaries, progress logs, and regular visits to a local health club. In a bungalowed suburb where employees come from old-fashioned Eastern European families, the same program falls flat. Why the different results? Because of the different preferences, values, and backgrounds of the employees, and also because of the different missions, values, and visions of the organizations and the kinds of people they tend to attract and retain.

The health care industry displays an intriguing paradox. Self-righteous MBAs are admonished to review an organization's financial statements for days just to leverage an additional two points off an investment. Yet, when it comes to human capital, motivation, pride, commitment, and a host of other intangible factors, that same organization treats all its employees alike. "We have a morale problem here" is how CEOs typically articulate a broad array of undifferentiated, intangible concerns. But not everyone in the organization may suffer from a morale problem; further, not everyone should be prodded to adopt the same solution.

The currently most popular form of generic change programs turns on compensation. Now viewed as the panacea for the nursing crisis, the idea that money buys happiness will soon find its way into recruitment and retention programs for medical technologists, family practitioners, pharmacists, and respiratory therapists. Unfortunately, this approach is an extension of a larger societal concept that views money as a one-way ticket to a better life. As experience demonstrates, however, throwing money at a personnel problem never solves it. Intangible problems such as lack of commitment cannot be solved by tangible inputs such as cash. In almost all cases, executives must instead attack the larger issues of organizational structure and make sure that people fit into a values context that promotes commitment and increases self-esteem.

One hospital CEO thought that he had solved his nurse retention problem by giving his nurses handsome raises. At one time, the hospital made money with a 65 percent occupancy rate, but now it needs more than 80 percent occupancy to meet its profitability goals. What will happen when the nurses' morale needs another boost and the hospital needs a 105 percent occupancy rate to turn a profit? You need not be an accountant to figure out that this CEO is caught in a powerful undertow. The message is simple: If you throw money at an intangible problem now, you will probably end up throwing more money at that same problem in the future. And employees may come to expect not only a decent wage but regular, generous increases as well. Satisfaction can be bought but commitment must be earned!

Beneath the Surface. If some health care executives try to fit every organizational recruit into the same bland uniform, others tiptoe on the surface of problems like mice on cotton. What they fail to take into account is that most organizations exist on three levels: the artifacts or "climate" level that is apparent to everyone, the values level that drives behavior, and the deep structure created by a mosaic of independent personalities. But why do some executives never delve below the first level? In most cases, it is easier to grapple with the more superficial issues related to job satisfaction. The question, What would it take to make you happy? usually elicits familiar answers: a child-care center, better food in the cafeteria, a more convenient parking place, or more pay. While these are important, they have less to do with building commitment than with job satisfaction. Commitment comes from engendering feelings of respect and providing chances to grow as a professional.

In contrast, consider the response provoked by these questions: What would increase your loyalty and commitment to this organization? What would it take to really "turn you on" to work? Few employees would mention the quality of the coffee, summertime baseball outings, or Christmas bonuses. Instead, if questioned in depth, they might talk about their desire to share tasks with other professionals and enrich their work life by learning new skills. Of course, none of these are easy solutions. You will not find them in the latest management best-seller because they come from the heart and soul of your employees. The problem is that soliciting employees' ideas takes time. Putting their ideas into practice takes even longer.

Is it any wonder therefore that many executives take the easy and most obvious way out? But if their analytical approach finds solutions only at the simplest level, they will get snared in a neverending struggle to make people happy. Failure is inevitable because, as noted before, employees' expectations begin to escalate. Because they are neither self-managed nor self-motivated, these individuals continually look to various kinds of satisfiers for compensation. A culture based almost entirely on external rewards will limit staff behavior. So what choice do staff members have but to ask for more and more?

In contrast, a strong, values-based culture defines the context for appropriate behavior. In a values-based culture, people focus on how their work contributes to the organization and how the organization improves personal feelings of worth. Remember that employees work to increase their psychic income. And the more they are treated like doormats, the more they want to be paid, because their only feelings of worth come from their paychecks.

The final question for executives in the course of analysis is this: Do we have the right people doing the right job at the right time? If you focus on the happiness quotient—on the satisfiers—people may be happy, but will not necessarily be committed to the organization. If you focus on matching core corporate values with employee values, however, staff will be both happy *and* committed.

Treating a troubled organization with special programs such as stress management seminars, employee service awards, and Christmas get-togethers at the president's house is like trying to treat cardiac disease exclusively with rest. The treatment has merit but is not sufficient. To recover completely, the heart patient needs a total life-style change brought about by changes in the way he eats, exercises, and manages stress. In the same way, the executive will never achieve success by investing in the management development "program of the month" and hiding behind the costly armor of new workbooks, videos, and overheads.

For leaders to change their organizations, they must be willing to take risks and be prepared for a long struggle. Leaders resist the temptation to delegate the task to a senior associate, vice-president of human resources, or even their favorite administrative assistant. A leader's chief task is to discover what it is that will energize the organization. No focused effects will occur without leadership, but the results will be worth the effort. Remember, culture drives behavior, and culture begins and ends with leadership.

Leaders are CEOs because they are *caring, empowering,* and *open.* Leaders create CEO employees who are *committed,* filled with *energy,* and quick to seize on *opportunities.* To determine if they have this kind of culture, leaders should ask themselves whether the following descriptions apply to them:

Caring: Do they regularly show employees that they care about them and the organization? Are they perceived as sincere? Are "managing by walking about" efforts viewed as management manipulation and empty rhetoric?

Empowering: What gives the work force a sense of power and mastery? Do employees feel free to explore new skills and knowledge areas? Are they encouraged to be innovative and take risks, even though they may fail at times?

Open: Have the leaders made themselves available and accessible? Do they listen to inarticulate frustrations and gripes as well as to carefully thought-out plans? Do they entertain and encourage dialogue? Do they allow the work force enough time to pursue new ideas? Are they empathetic?

After addressing these issues, leaders should consider the impact of their behavior on their followers.

Committed: To what extent have the members of the work force become more committed to the organization? Does their concern for the organization outweigh their egoistic concerns? What would cause them to change employers?

Energetic: Do members of the work force feel liberated enough to experiment and try new things? To what extent are they rewarded for innovations and experimentation? Or is innovation thwarted by cliches such as "incremental change?" Are people praised or punished for criticizing current programs and suggesting better ways?

Open to Change: How many unsolicited, new ideas appeared on their desks in the past month? What evidence is there that if a new idea or concept is introduced, it will be acknowledged, reviewed, and evaluated seriously? Do people understand the process for introducing new ideas into the organization? Is the work force on the alert to find out about the innovations of competitors, colleagues, and other industries?

Many years ago, a leading professor and management consultant created a strategy called management by objectives (MBO). People were designated good managers according to how well they fulfilled predetermined goals and objectives, and managers were judged very superior, superior, average, or unsatisfactory according to how easy it was for their boss to check the list of objectives and document compliance with them.

Now, however, the acronym MBO can have a new, more

enlightened meaning: managing behavioral opportunities. Leaders must do more than fulfill broad strategic goals and tactical objectives. They must also behave in ways that develop the responses they want from their followers. An executive must ask: Is the work force committed, energized, and ready to seize new opportunities? Or is it frustrated, disenfranchised, detached, and content to maintain the status quo for fear of doing something wrong? If the answer to the second question is yes, there probably is a long way to go before this executive becomes a leader.

Fixing Blame. In analyzing an organization, some executives find it easy to fix blame on "the other guy." After all, if a person can place the responsibility on someone else, he can remain innocent—at least for awhile. For example, if an executive can convince others that most of the problems at his hospital are the work of troublesome, greedy physicians, he can then disclaim all responsibility for causing the problems or for finding solutions to them. Furthermore, he can minimize his own sense of failure or disappointment because the problem never had anything to do with him. After all, "It was those doctors. If they had the sense to stick to the business of practicing medicine," he tells board members, "this could have been avoided."

At one time or another, we have all played this game. We do it with such ease and innocence that it is often difficult to catch ourselves. Consider these examples: A student fails an exam because "the teacher didn't explain the material clearly." A woman remains overweight because "this situation is driving me crazy. I have to eat to forget it." An employee is continually tardy because "I have so much work that I am always tired and wake up late."

To rely on these excuses and pass blame on to others is very human. But executives who engage in this behavior on a regular basis are executives in name only. Why? Because they refuse to accept that they may be part of the problem. More importantly, they have the responsibility to create positive change.

Leaders should ask themselves: Is it always someone else's problem? Do I tend to use phrases such as: "That's a decision you'll have to make for yourself." "The problem with those people is that they won't change." "They don't understand what we're doing over here." "Why can't they get with the program?" "We need people who can take this organization in the right direction." "I'm a good leader, I wish I had better followers."

If the problem is always with a person, department, organization, or entity that is supposedly outside the executive's control, then something is seriously wrong with his approach to leadership. If replacing employees, restructuring the organization, remodeling his office is his treatment of choice, then perhaps he needs to spend more time reflecting on his own behavior. Perhaps he should ask himself these questions: When I accuse people of not wanting to change, have I really developed an adequate rationale for change? Do people feel secure and protected enough to make the change? Do they understand the direction and consequences of the change? If they don't understand the grand design for the organization, does this mean that communication channels are inadequate? How can rumors and misperceptions be controlled and corrected? What steps can be taken to make people feel more invested and involved?

If a leader is willing to take ownership of behavior, she will immediately notice a difference in the quality and character of her language. Ineffective leaders often become the victims of language, drowning in the latest management lingo about "self-starters" who can "hit the deck running" or mired in flowery cliches about the organization's being a "real family." Most often, however, they are obsessed with what was or what might have been and constantly lament, "we should have done this last year" or "I wish the government would stop taking advantage of us."

Effective leaders take a different tack. Instead of going on nostalgic journeys through decades past or touring tomorrowland, they use language to assume more responsibility and to take aggressive action. Rather than trying to fix blame or spending their time in a fantasy world, effective leaders focus on what is happening here and now and seek out the meaning of events and situations. They are likely to say, "There's very little we can do to change this decision. Things aren't the way they used to be and we're going to have to accept that. But what we can do is create a more effective organization, and I'm going to make sure that people here get all the support they need to do it."

Leaders calm the troubled waters of organizations by their

willingness to climb to the highest point of the mountain and see if the sun is peeking from behind a cloud or if storm clouds are on the horizon. They know that, as the environment changes, the options for action also change. These days, health care needs more leaders who offer a mountain-top perspective. Without it, executives will continue to narrowly analyze staff motivation as a compensation problem and ignore more basic issues. For example, to the question, How are we going to deliver quality health care to patients if key staff are no longer committed, the answer must be: Change the organization and clarify the roles and responsibilities of workers. Without an elevated perspective, executives will continue to seek the quick fix—which only serves as a temporary opiate.

Chapter Six

Assessment:
Conducting an Inventory of the Organization and Yourself

Leaders should survey the organization's environment to determine the readiness of staff for an assessment. They should ask questions such as these:

- How am I planning to use this assessment? Is it a carrot or a club? Am I secretly hoping to flush out troublemakers and punish the guilty? Or am I committed to using this assessment as the first step in building a more effective organization?
- Does this assessment have a clear-cut context and purpose? Have I communicated this context and purpose to every key member in the organization?
- Have I already fixed in my mind the nature of this organization's problems? Or am I truly open to this assessment? Am I prepared to deal with the data—no matter how negative or threatening they may be?
- Are my expectations for the assessment realistic, specific, and attainable?
- Have I carefully identified the recipients and users of the data? Are they committed to the process and to the outcome of the assessment? How will I involve them in designing the instrument, analyzing the data, and communicating the results?

73

- Have I explored how the data from the assessment will be an-alyzed and communicated? What channels of communication will be most effective?
- Have I taken the time to deal candidly with peoples' fears and concerns? Have I provided adequate assurance that no one will get hurt in the process? Do people understand that the goal of the process is not to fix blame or build secret personnel files, but to create a better organization?
- What assurances do I have that the data will be valid and reli-able? Does the instrument have a good track record in the health care industry? Is it reliable? If we were repeatedly to administer the same instrument, would it produce the same results?
- In sum, am I fully prepared to answer these questions about the assessment: Why are we carrying out the assessment? What are we going to assess? How should we structure this assessment? What will we do with the data?

On the Road to Assessment

As the assessment process begins, there are several things to keep in mind:

1. Instruments that are little more than Dr. Feelgood "cli-mate" or satisfaction surveys should be avoided. Worrying about job satisfaction—how happy people are—will do little to enhance the likelihood that they will remain with the organization. But focusing on commitment factors—such as recognition, self-management, and affiliation—increases the chance that employees will want to stay. If commitment drives a leader's professional life, he is likely to respond to an alluring job offer with, "Thanks, but I'm really involved here. I believe in this place. They've helped me through some hard times and I want to see this thing through."

Employee attitudes are important, but attitudes alone will never give a total picture of life in the organization. Nor will a highly quantitative, productivity profile necessarily lead the way to future success. The starting point of assessment is in values—who one is and what one believes in. These are the convictions that drive behavior. A disservice is performed if productivity is measured with-out looking at why people are unproductive. No contribution is made if attitudes are measured without looking at the values that support them.

2. The assessment focuses cannot do it all. Diagnosis, by itself, does not solve the problem. Insight must be followed by action. Executives often think that they can fix human behavior as easily as a glazier can fix a broken window. Unfortunately, this is almost never the case. Typically, it takes the same amount of time to fix a problem as it did to create it.

Behavior changes slowly, except in the case of trauma. Of course, pain, shock, and trauma can be created by using terror tactics, but such strategies will not be worth the effort in the long term. Change that follows trauma usually carries a heavy price tag. Ultimately, people will regress, rebel, or even engage in sabotage.

The primary purpose of assessment is to determine how well people fit within the organization. So if an employee, physician, or board member has a personal history that directly conflicts with the organization, resist the temptation to put the two together and then try to work a miracle. Leaders have better ways to invest their time, talent, and energy.

3. The leader needs to be aware of the history and tradition of assessment in the organization. A CEO who wanted to retain control of every management decision outraged his employees when he announced an upcoming assessment of the organization. Insulted and threatened by the process, employees viewed the assessment exercise as an opportunity to settle some old scores with the boss. They used the assessment not only to communicate a message but also to take revenge for the irritating way in which he meddled in their affairs.

In assessing the organization, a leader should be aware of people's attitudes toward and experiences with assessment tools used in the past. Typically, most people wince at the word *assessment*. Like the student who is unprepared for a test, the reluctant employee will do everything from lashing out at the boss to spreading rumors about how "test" results will be used. On an even more basic level, most people like to think of themselves as unique or special. How could anyone reduce who they are and what they do to a survey, they wonder. The reality, of course, is that most human behavior—especially in the workplace—is fairly predictable.

4. The leader ties the assessment to the mission, values, and vision of the organization. For what purpose does our organization exist? What do we believe in? Where are we headed? These questions are the essence of each phase of the assessment, analysis, and action process. If an executive engages in casual, weekly chats on the topic of motivation with one of her managers, the information garnered is no doubt rich in interesting data. However, one issue will remain: What is the context for these data? What is their meaning? How does this information and data relate to the organization's mission, vision, and values?

5. The leader focuses on the deeper motivational values that drive behavior. Accountants and math wizards may disagree, but it is still relatively easy to lie with statistics. If employees are encouraged to be open and candid about what they think of the organization, will it really make a difference? The result will be a confused patchwork of euphemisms, cliches, and mild suggestions about "things that might be worked on." In developing any assessment, you must first answer one question: Am I measuring attitudes or am I measuring behavior? Despite the lip service paid to "the magic of language," words are cheap in our society. Attention should focus on behavior. What people do defines who they are.

6. Assessment is the first step before taking action. Sixty pounds overweight and a smoker more than twenty years, Myra continually cancelled appointments with her physician. Finally, she admitted, "If I don't hear him tell me what's wrong, I don't have to deal with it." At least in the short-term, Myra functions better by avoiding diagnosis and assessment of something she already understands on an intuitive level.

Many executives—especially those at the helm of dysfunctional organizations—are surprisingly like Myra. By avoiding the assessment process, they postpone confrontation with the truth. At least for a short time, they can hold fast to the status quo. And in a worst-case scenario, they can transfer blame to others. "Fix our managers," they say to consultants. But what happens when the consultant follows senior management directives and salvages or redirects only the most troublesome units? All too frequently, one unit moves off in one direction, while others remain stagnant or head the opposite way.

7. The assessment should focus on people. It is people on whom an assessment should concentrate. Unfortunately, most executives look at organizational artifacts such as policies, procedures, and plans, even though written policies and procedures are no guarantee of organizational effectiveness. The Joint Commission on Accreditation of Healthcare Organizations, for example, has recently shifted its attention to organizational intangibles such as leadership, mission, and change.

8. Assessment is an ongoing program—not just a component of the annual performance appraisal. In most industries, people are assessed in annual evaluations that have more to do with anniversary dates than with behavior and performance. Typically, the principle of recency dominates: People are often evaluated on the basis of the accomplishments they recorded and the mistakes they made in the sixty days immediately before the evaluation. Moreover, most executives feel compelled to find something wrong with their employees. No one could be that good, they reason. There's no such thing as a very superior rating. As a result, executives often dish out an equal measure of carrots and sticks.

In the worst case, these evaluations deflate and demotivate employees. If you find this hard to believe, answer this question: When was the last time an annual evaluation motivated you to greater productivity and excellence? Ask the same question of your colleagues and you will probably discover that evaluations often diminish performance. Not only does preevaluation anxiety reduce productivity, but, in many cases, employees will be tortured by self-doubts after an evaluation: Why am I here? What am I doing? I'm giving the best years of my life to this organization and what am I getting in return?

During an annual evaluation, a nursing director was told, "Some people around here don't think you're a very good manager." "What do you mean?" she asked. "Give me some examples." "Well, I really can't say," the superior replied. "I just want you to know that there's a perception." Three hours after the evaluation, the director felt as though she had been torpedoed. Unfortunately, her attitude toward herself and her work came to be shaped almost exclusively by the comments of her boss.

Or consider the manager of dietary services who is verbally

drawn and quartered in her vice-president's office, only to hear him close the conversation with a wink, a smile, and the words, "We really like having you around here." If workers are labeled good one day and bad the next, of if they are labeled as both good and bad in the same conversation, what will they believe and whom will they trust? Bewildered and irritated, these employees typically become less effective in their jobs and avoid contact with their unpredictable superiors.

What, then, is the ideal? A healthy organization prepares people to engage in self-evaluation and self-motivation within ninety days of their hire dates. It is made clear to them that behavior A is productive and valuable to the organization, whereas behavior B is destructive and should be avoided. In this scheme, annual evaluations become nothing more than a tool to record accomplishments of the previous year and prepare goals for the coming year.

9. People need to be reassured. They need permission to express their beliefs in person or on paper with no fear of reprisal. When an organizational assessment is scheduled, leaders realize that people may be on the defensive. They take the time to let people know that they understand the reasons for their defensiveness. Most importantly, they make it clear to employees that the purpose of assessment is not to weed out undesirables. The purpose of the assessment is to focus the purpose of the organization and the work values of the employees. Given that purpose, the roles and contributions of employees can be clarified.

10. Assessment and evaluation must be distinguished from each other. Assessment involves the collection of data while evaluation involves judgment. In most cases, judgments, decisions, statements, and evaluations should be buttressed by data, evidence, and supporting material. Even if statistics are not available, the main points can be clarified and explained by example, quotation, illustration, or even analogy. Take the case in which a nursing director is informed that some people perceive her as a less than ideal manager. She requests data but never receives specific feedback. Contrast that evaluation with one in which her superior states, "That report came in by 4:00 P.M.; it should have been here by 10:00 A.M."

11. Even when the data have been gathered, judgment on the organization must still be suspended. Despite the claims of pop

management books, there are no good or bad cultures. In World War II General George Patton created a highly effective culture for the mission he had to accomplish. In the same way, Mother Theresa has the most effective culture for her mission. Both General Patton and Mother Theresa are regarded as highly successful, charismatic leaders, but they had fundamentally different missions. Cultures, therefore, are neither inherently good nor bad. (Some, of course, can become pathological and destructive, usually because of an underground network of subcultures that wage war with each other.) Through the assessment process, data can be collected on the strength of the organization's culture. Judgment should be reserved until then.

12. The roles of those who are to be assessed and those who are to use the data need to be identified. There must also be a clear understanding of who will design the assessment instrument, who will make decisions about the questions, who will receive the survey, and who will ultimately use the data.

13. The assessment should be conducted and processed by outside facilitators, since it is very difficult to administer an assessment of one's own organization. Is the president of a financially troubled organization really the best person to lead a management/ board retreat on turnaround strategies? Unfortunately, many executives are slow to accept the necessity of consultants who deal with human capital. They pay $300 per hour to attorneys without a second thought; they bring in accountants when only a minor variation is uncovered in financial statements. And when a new building is needed, few executives sit down on the weekend with a book on architectural design. Nevertheless, these same executives often assume that they can easily understand human motivation.

14. Leaders must ask what their personal motivations are for conducting the assessment. Inevitably, people will ask, Why are we doing this anyway? An answer must be forthcoming. If the assessment is meant to round up winners and losers, the more savvy people in the organization will sense that. In the end, considerable money and time will have been expended on what amounts to a witch hunt. The more serious consequence is that the organization may end up more troubled than it was before the assessment.

In the same way, the barriers to assessment must be confronted. As mentioned before, many executives hold back on assessment out of fear of what it may uncover. As one cautious CEO asked, "What if I find out that morale is low?" But an assessment tool would do nothing more than quantify the situation so that he could take action. Unfortunately, some CEOs prefer to serve as caretakers of dysfunctional organizations rather than confront the truth and do the hard work needed to manage change.

Assessment is admittedly difficult. It means that the government, physicians, fluoridated water, employers, Wall Street, the crumbling public educational system, or some other societal ill can no longer be blamed. The fact is that the destiny of an organization and its people is in the leader's hands. In the course of an assessment it may even be discovered that the reluctance to assess the organization is rooted in the leader's philosophy of human nature. If so, she must be brutally frank with herself. Does she believe that people need to be whipped or they won't perform well? Does she see employees as little more than interchangeable parts in the management machine? Does she look upon the new-fangled theories about human capital as mindless drivel?

In sum, data collection tools, as well as the spirit or attitude with which the assessment is conducted, should be approached cautiously. Most of all, every effort should be made to turn what could be a boring, tedious schoolroom exercise into an opportunity. Quite simply, conducting an assessment should be seen as a way to produce a more effective organization.

Selecting an Assessment Tool

Once the organization is ready to begin the assessment process, it must choose an appropriate instrument. The following instrument contains material from the Healthcare Organizational Assessment Survey designed by MetriTech, Inc. (pp. 3-7). The Healthcare Organizational Assessment Survey (Larry A. Braskamp, Ph.D., and Martin L. Maehr, Ph.D.) is copyright © 1986 by Metri-Tech, Inc., 111 North Market Street, Champaign, IL. (217) 398-4868. Reproduced by permission. This 200-item survey uses *The Motivation Factor: A Theory of Personal Investment* as the basis for its design. It assesses the four dimensions of recognition, accomplishment, power, and affiliation according to how people perceive themselves, their jobs, and the organization.

Recognition

Person: How important are financial rewards and acknowledgments from others?

Job: Do employees receive extra benefits for doing good work?

Organization: Do people believe the organization does a good job of rewarding the achievements and contributions of its employees?

If recognition is a strong value, people give positive responses to the following statements:

- Employees in this organization receive a lot of attention.
- In this organization, they make me feel like a winner.
- This organization allows me to do those things that I find personally satisfying.
- There are many incentives to work hard.

Accomplishment

Person: How much do people strive for excellence and how much do they enjoy and value challenging and exciting work?

Job: To what extent do they strive for excellence in what they do? Is this job an exciting and challenging one?

Organization: Does this organization emphasize excellence in products and services?

If accomplishment is a strong value in your organization, people will respond positively to the following statements:

- I am encouraged to make suggestions about how we can be more effective.
- Around here, we are encouraged to try new things.

- In this organization, we are given a great deal of freedom to carry out our work.
- If someone has a good idea, invention, or project, management will listen and support it.

Power

> *Person:* To what degree do employees compete with one another to gain authority and to advance within the organization?
>
> *Job:* Can I influence others through this job?
>
> *Organization:* Does this organization create an environment in which conflict and competition are assumed and expected?

If power is a strong value in your organization, people will respond positively to the following statements:

- Successful people are those who like to win.
- I emerged as the leader of my group.
- People seek me out for advice.
- Competition among different work groups is actively encouraged.

Affiliation

> *Person:* How important are showing concern and affection to others and making sacrifices to help others develop?
>
> *Job:* Does this job help others?
>
> *Organization:* Is the organization one that emphasizes mutual support, open communication, sharing of information, and caring for each individual?

If affiliation is a strong value, people will respond positively to the following statements:

- In this organization, they really care about me as a person.
- We are treated like adults in this organization.
- In this organization, there is respect for each individual worker.

- I am involved in decisions that directly affect my work in this organization.

   For each of the four values, the focus should be on three factors: the person, the job, and the organization. To assess these factors, employees should be asked to respond to the following series of statements by noting if they (1) strongly agree, (2) agree, (3) are uncertain, (4) disagree, or (5) strongly disagree.

   The first set of questions is meant to elicit information about the personality of the employee:

- I enjoy completing many easy tasks rather than just a few difficult ones.
- I pay little attention to the interests of people around me.
- I want recognition for what I do.
- I emerged as a leader in my group.

   In a similar way, employees' reactions to their present job or position in the organization can be evaluated by asking them to choose an answer that completes the following statement: My Present Job Provides Opportunities

- to show my competence and ability.
- to help people directly.
- to receive recognition for my work.
- to hire and fire employees.

   Finally, it can be determined how people feel about the organization by asking them to react to the following statements:

- My co-workers and I work well together.
- I feel I get sufficient pay for the work I do.
- I have the opportunity to do good work here and thus advance myself.
- I have a sense of loyalty to this place.

   Responses to these and similar questions provide three outcome measurements—strength of culture, job satisfaction, and organizational commitment, which together form the bottom line of human capital.

Strength of Culture (Balance Sheet). How strong is the organization's culture? Do employees believe that the organization has done a good job of defining and communicating its mission? Do they see the organization as having a clear sense of direction (vision)? Do people understand what is expected of them (values)? If the culture is strong, employees see their organization as having a clear set of norms and and a strong sense of direction. They know what the organization stands for and what really counts. Agreement on values is pervasive and deep. Each employee has a strong sense of ownership in what happens around him or her.

Job Satisfaction (Profit/Loss). How satisfied are people with their work, pay, promotion opportunities, supervision, and co-workers? When people experience job satisfaction, they answer the question, Do you enjoy your job? with an emphatic yes. If people are committed to an organization, they tend to enjoy their jobs. But it does not necessarily follow that someone who is satisfied with his or her job is committed to the organization. Although satisfaction might not predict commitment, commitment predicts satisfaction.

Commitment (Net Worth). Viewed another way, commitment—not satisfaction—predicts retention, and commitment comes from shared values, meaning, loyalty, pride, and ownership. Hospitals with strong cultures enjoy high levels of commitment among their workers. If people commit themselves to an organization, they believe in it and understand it. Only when an organization has a defined mission, internalized values, and a clear vision are employees likely to say, "Now that we understand what we're about, we know how we fit in and we won't leave here."

Culture, commitment, and satisfaction can be analyzed for the organization as well as for distinct subgroups within it—for example, the senior management team, board members, medical staff leadership, department heads, and support staff. Total organizational scores provide a good starting point, but viewing the scores according to subgroups will both pinpoint areas of strengths that can be used to better the organization and identify those weaknesses that may require special attention when instituting any kind of managed change program.

Assessing Leadership Skills

The period just after completion of the organizational assessment may be the perfect time for the leader to further assess his leadership skills. The leader should rate himself on each of the issues listed below. In each case he should describe his typical behaviors and actions, as well as how people are affected by them. A leader should pose two questions: What is my standard operating procedure? Does it motivate or demotivate people?

Structure. How is work structured? Does the structure liberate people and make them more productive? Or does it constrain and demoralize people?

Feedback. What kind of feedback do people receive? In what form and through what vehicles? To what extent is the feedback constructive, positive, and motivating? To what extent is it negative? How often do you hear people say, "You never get a thank you around here. They never appreciate what you do"? To what degree are people affected by the absence of positive feedback? Are you guilty of delivering mixed messages that confuse and traumatize people?

Productivity. How is productivity defined and measured in this organization? To what extent is it guilty of a desire to reduce all performance to "standards?" Are individuals who can produce financial gains or cost savings rewarded more consistently than those who make significant intangible contributions? What is the organization's concept of a "productive employee" and how does that person differ from a "busy employee?"

Failure. To what extent does this organization encourage risk taking and tolerate—even accept—failure? How are people encouraged to take risks? What kinds of safety nets or parachutes are provided? When people failed in the past, how were they treated? How are people treated when they succeed?

Accountability. How are people held accountable for their performance? To what extent are people given clear expectations as well as opportunities to "stretch?" Are people allowed to pass the buck and blame others for their failures or is self-management the norm?

Communication. When decisions are made, how are they shared with the organization? To what extent are people given the opportunity for serious input? Is criticism tolerated and even encouraged? Or are outspoken employees punished as disruptive troublemakers? How are disputes or conflicts resolved? Is silence interpreted as compliance/support?

Ownership. To what extent do people feel invested in the organization? Are they able to decide independently and take action, or do they always have to appeal to higher authority? How are autonomy and personal growth encouraged? To what extent are people encouraged to give positive feedback to themselves and others? Or do people depend exclusively on their superiors or on financial rewards for validation of self-worth?

Recognition. How is recognition tied to values-based behavior? Are people rewarded through promotions and compensation as well as through service pins. Are they rewarded for values-based, mission-driven, and team-oriented behavior? Or are rewards consistently given to hard-nosed, bottom-line contributors?

Values. Are values instilled at all levels of this organization? If so, through what vehicles? Do people understand the values of this organization and how they can be translated into behavior? Are the values felt "in the gut?"

Unfortunately, many instruments designed to assess leadership measure only satisfiers and dissatisfiers. Independent of an organization's context, satisfiers mean little. Many health care executives who have risen to top spots in religious institutions would probably last about three weeks in investor-owned systems. In the same way, an aggressive, financially oriented MBA might grow frustrated and impatient with an organization that began each day in meditation and prayer. Although these executives might have similar personalities, their behavior is guided by different beliefs and values.

Leadership theories often focus solely on what leaders do and ignore what potential followers need. This is a mistake. Leadership must concern itself both with actions and the impact of those actions on others. Leadership involves not only action and quantifiable results but also the spirit that is developed and built within the organization. Leadership is more than a matter of new and better programs and services; it also encompasses the values and beliefs that are integrated into new projects. Leadership starts with what a person does and ends with the effects of those actions on the people who are expected to follow.

All too often, executives embrace the latest best-selling business book as a cure for their own organization's ills. Although they see promise in the maneuvers of a Lee Iacocca, a Sam Walton, or a John Scully, they often discover that imitation—while it may be a sincere form of flattery—usually has limited impact. As the fumbling successor to the CEO of a major health care system once said, "I don't know what's wrong. I'm doing everything he did." In making that statement, he was missing a crucial point: Plans, procedures, and policies were essential ingredients to his predecessor's success, but even more important were that individual's values and the spirit he infused into his followers.

Consider the health care executive who has read every book published on leadership in the last five years. He understands the magic of one-minute interactions, management by walking around, and even dressing for success. Although he appears to do everything right, nothing works. Why? Because he never assimilated the philosophies and principles that undergird innovative organizations and drive entrepreneurial executives. As a result, he comes off like a used car salesman in a pin-striped suit. He uses all the right words and gestures, but no one believes him.

Leadership is a by-product of what a person believes about the people whom she wants to turn into followers. If she looks upon these individuals as valuable human beings and effective workers with unlimited potential, her role will become that of facilitator, servant, enabler. A leader's task is to motivate people by making them feel positive about themselves, their performance, and the organization. A leader views people as partners and associates in a collective quest.

The ultimate goals of assessment are self-monitoring and ownership of behavior (accountability). A person who is unable to monitor herself necessarily depends on outside authority for direction. "I don't know what to do," is her typical response. "I'll talk to my boss." In organizations with strong leadership, something else happens. Everyone in the organization—regardless of position—learns to make decisions that benefit the organization because everyone knows what the organization stands for. Everyone feels confident and has access to the information necessary to make decisions consistent with the aims of the organization. Confident that failure will not result in painful reprisals, individuals feel free to disregard the limitations of a specific job description.

Self-managed, motivated employees communicate their enthusiasm for their work and their organization. Such people live service. And today, service is the difference between success and failure.

No matter what the industry, these are the individuals who are truly priceless. They may not have college degrees or upper-middle-class backgrounds, but they know how to make decisions and take action. Because their motivation comes from within—because they are confident in their decision making—they are ready to accept responsibility. They do not respond with "I'll have to check on that," "That's not my area," or "You need to talk to someone else." They feel good about what they do with and for others and become increasingly confident of their ability to perform new and challenging tasks. In the same way, they feel increasingly committed to the organization that helps to nurture their growth and development. They feel secure because they know that the leader believes in their competence, and they are proud of the contribution that they make to the organization's success.

These individuals are effective because they function in a context that is defined, clarified, and reinforced by the highest levels of the organization. They know who they are and how their work contributes to the greater good of the organization. In addition, they know their limits and where they may need to ask for support or advice. They spend few sleepless nights anticipating shocks in their annual performance reviews because they understand where and how they excelled and where and how they missed the mark.

At twenty-nine, Art was a battle-scarred veteran of five years as an associate administrator at a large urban teaching institution where mistakes were seen as the result of serious character defects. In his first few months in a new organization, Art continually asked for permission, direction, and guidance. Finally, his new boss took him aside and said, "If you don't make at least five mistakes a day, you're not working. The only real mistake you can make is not to try new things." At first Art was skeptical and confused, but gradually he came into his own. Freed from the bondage of a punitive organization, he no longer had to do Monday morning battle with his superior. Because he felt liberated to explore new areas, work became its own reward. For the first time in his professional life, Art knew that he was doing an effective job because he had the confidence to evaluate his actions and the results they produced.

Art's case is not an unusual one. Many people who go down for the count in organizations that pay lip service to innovation are able to restore their faith in themselves when they move to a new environment. In contrast, managers on the receiving end of an unceasing barrage of mixed messages often find it difficult to give their friends odds on whether they will be fired or promoted within the next sixty days. As a result, they typically withdraw from co-workers, refuse new commitments, and, like an airplane over a crowded airport, go into a holding pattern. Utterly dependent on the feedback of troubled superiors, they are more apt to atrophy than to grow.

In effective organizations, people are given plenty of leeway to achieve the organization's vision. Like the person controlling the rudder of a sailboat, they know their destination and what they need to do to get there. They make good decisions because they have the confidence to review a situation and pass judgment. Although they may sometimes take over management responsibilities, they also understand their limits. If a severe storm is brewing on the horizon, that sailor at the rudder knows enough to check with the captain.

Chapter Seven

Analysis:
Focusing on the Target

Leaders understand that if data are to motivate staff, they must be converted to meaningful information. Interpretation and judgment provide the bridge between assessment and analysis, between data and information. Interpretation means describing the data in specific, concrete, and objective terms (for example, "motivation is increasing in operations"; "satisfaction is down in the emergency room"; or "commitment is up with the surgeons"). Interpretation tells us what the numbers say. Judgment tells us how fast we can go, how much we can expect, and our overall vision/goal/ objectives.

Analysis is fundamentally different from assessment. During assessment, behavior is converted into numbers. In analysis, leaders try to evaluate the numbers. Analysis is nothing more than judging the numbers to be "good" or "bad." If you discover that your blood pressure is 190 over 150, it means little until your physician tells you, "That's high." The physician has analyzed the numbers, given them meaning, and made a judgment. Leadership requires you to accept the responsibility of evaluation and to help staff understand the context of your decisions.

Typically, analysis makes use of words such as *good, reliable, effective,* and *worthwhile.* Evaluation is evident in these statements: "Our greatest asset is our nursing staff." "This survey received a better response rate than the last one." "The level of participation in that program is disappointing." "Morale is low this month." All these statements involve judgments based on data. They go beyond a description of what is occurring to an assertion of whether or not something is good or bad, harmful or beneficial, negative or positive. Leaders always anchor judgments in the organization's culture. Remember, there are no good or bad cultures, and judgments about goodness or badness can only be made in the context of the corporate culture. Judging data in context is the essence of analysis and your key function as a health care leader committed to organizational change. Culture-based analysis is the foundation of all manged change programs.

Effective Organizations

The effective health care organization is characterized by five factors: high quality, high commitment, high patient satisfaction, high market share, and high profit. When these factors are present, the culture is strong, change is being managed well, and there is a good sense of teamwork. The more effective your organization, the more these factors will increase. However, if you notice that quality, commitment, patient satisfaction, profit, and market share are on the downswing, you will want to introduce the questions, How do we become a more effective organization? What aspect of our culture changed and why? Why did commitment weaken? Did the organization fail to offer enough recognition to good employees? Why did people come to feel less attached to their jobs?

Take time out to analyze the effectiveness of your organization by asking these questions:

- How personally invested are your employees? Are there reasons to be concerned about their level of commitment?
- What is the most effective part of your organization? What is driving the corporate culture?
- Is your vision of the organization clear to your employees? Do they all know the direction you are taking the company? Have you clarified their role in achieving this direction?
- How successful will you be in achieving your tangible objec-

tives by means of the intangible motivational aspects revealed by your assessment?

- How would you change your profile? What would be ideal for the support staff, medical staff, board of trustees, professional staff, and management team. For example, would you want to become more risk-taking and entrepreneurial or would you want more teamwork and bottom-up decision making?
- If you need to strengthen your culture, what values should you emphasize?

Financial audits are used to identify business strengths and weaknesses. In a somewhat similar way, culture audits are used to isolate effective practices that correspond to the values of the organization and to identify the areas that must be emphasized if a positive corporate culture is to be maintained. The use of culture audits is tied to the analysis and interpretation of assessment data. The leader must bring all these factors to bear when developing a plan of action, and the following section provides a complete list of the audit factors to be used in identifying areas of change.

Mission/Strategic Planning

1. We have a set of long-range goals that we continually revise.
2. We use these long-range goals as a basis for hiring new people.
3. We distribute revisions of goals to our staff.
4. We discuss our mission statement at least twice a year.
5. We spend more time on long-range plans than on short-term solutions.

Socialization

1. I often hear stories about the contributions of our leaders and staff.
2. This organization is never dull or unexciting.
3. Leaders in the organization know how to get the employees to follow them.
4. We have social events in which we talk about the accomplishments of the organization.

5. Fellow employees take a new person to lunch on his or her first day at work.
6. We have parties to help new employees get to know their fellow workers better.
7. We recognize special events such as birthdays.
8. I often hear others speak of our organization as one big family.

Selection

1. People who work here must go through a thorough screening process to determine whether their personal values match corporate values.
2. Job roles are made explicit to each applicant.
3. Teamwork expectations are explained in order to screen out anyone who would not work well with others.

Standards/Expectations

1. Expectations about what and how much they will have to do are made clear to staff members in writing.
2. Employees are able to see how individual goals enhance the goals of the organization.
3. The organization has clear standards of performance, and those who do not meet them are helped with extra training.
4. If, after help, an employee does not meet corporate expectations, he or she is released from the organization.
5. If the expectations held by a staff and its supervisor do not agree, everyone feels free to discuss the problem openly.

Performance Appraisal

1. All employees work with their supervisors to define how to perform their duties and what they should be accomplishing.
2. Supervisors provide routine and frequent feedback.
3. All staff members have a say in how much they are to accomplish.
4. People who work here say that they would like more relevant and immediate information on how well they are doing.
5. Evaluation of work is very informal.
6. Evaluation only happens when a decision about promotion is needed.

7. Evaluation of work may include discussion about how to improve.
8. Supervisors always share work evaluations.

Team Work

1. We structure goals so that we can work together in teams.
2. Groups are rewarded as a unit when they are successful.
3. Groups share the responsibility of determining how to proceed to get work done.
4. We think in terms of group projects rather than individual assignments.

Participation in Management

1. The lines of authority in this organization are clear.
2. Everyone in the organization can take on almost any role since titles and positions mean little.
3. Before we make a decision or establish a policy, everyone who will be affected by it is consulted.
4. Employee participation in decision making is very high.
5. Many people review designs and plans before we implement them.
6. We hold special retreats to discuss the future of our organization.
7. Expectations for performance in this organization are clearly defined.
8. Rules and regulations are values based and internalized.
9. Our rules and regulations never get in the way of productivity.
10. We are known as a company with very little bureaucracy.

Communication Networks

1. Management promotes open communication among all units of the organization.
2. Staff meetings are held at least biweekly.
3. Communication in the organization is very informal.
4. House organs are used to communicate policies and practices.
5. All managers have an open-door policy.
6. Employees can go around their immediate supervisor if they have a problem.

7. Upper-level management sponsors lunches and open meetings to hear the concerns of the employees.

Career Succession/Advancement

1. Everyone is in charge of his or her own future in this organization.
2. Everyone is encouraged to grow professionally and to become a better team player.
3. There are many avenues for advancement in this organization.
4. Career counseling and advice are available.
5. Everyone can talk confidentially with those in human resources about the probability of advancing in the organization.

Organizational Adaptability

1. This organization makes changes quickly to meet increasing demands.
2. Everyone is very concerned about how others view our services.
3. We are continually doing market surveys to learn how to best meet the wants and needs of our customers.
4. We are continually experimenting with new programs and approaches to make our services better.
5. We are encouraged to take risks.
6. We work closely with our customers so that we can provide services that fit their needs and wants.
7. We are concerned about how our best clients view us.
8. We make it a point to listen carefully to what our customers and clients want from us.

Organizational Structure

1. We believe in adaptability and thus are always ready to reorganize.
2. We have a flat arrangement of positions and roles within the organization: little bureaucracy, few layers of management, and decision making close to those serving customers.
3. In this organization employees are put into small units that

have the freedom to do things the way the unit team thinks they should be done.

4. There are few layers of management in this organization.
5. In this organization the emphasis is on keeping the work units small and flexible.
6. To solve special problems we establish informal ad hoc task forces.
7. Every person in the organization is free to suggest new ideas and solutions to problems.
8. We emphasize the importance of each role within a team and spell out what is expected of the person in that role.

Recognition Practices

1. We have a parking spot for the employee of the month.
2. We have recognition dinners at least once a year.
3. We publish the pictures of those named employees of the month.
4. We have a policy of writing letters and notes to those who have done outstanding work.
5. There is a section in our house organ that deals with recognition of employees.
6. *All* recognition is based on team contributions to achieving the organization's vision within the context of our core values.

Financial Incentives/Salary Program

1. Exceptional teams can get bonuses.
2. Salary increases are based on team performance rather than on longevity.

Audit relationships show the causes of and barriers to building committed followers. Audits also show the variances in the strength of the organization's culture among different work groups. These variances will pinpoint areas where managed change is most feasible. It should be reiterated that there are no absolute right or wrong analyses. The important thing is to define those values that the organization emphasizes and to determine whether employees' values are in harmony with them.

Here are the essentials of how to build a positive corporate culture. A strong culture exists when (1) employees view the organization as having a clear set of values and a sense of direction, (2) employee values and organizational values converge, (3) commitment is high and jobs are challenging, (4) employees work cooperatively to achieve the organization's vision because they feel ownership of and pride in the success of the organization, (5) employees are encouraged to take risks and are rewarded for contributions to their team, and (6) the emphasis is on the human capital of the organization.

A Case Study

The following discussion explores how Elizabethtown University Hospital Rehabilitation Center in Elizabethtown, Pennsylvania, used assessment and analysis to develop specific change programs to enhance the corporate culture. The leadership team of Jeffrey Norman, which included Marie Zannotti, James Rohacek, Mary Ann Whinnerling, and Ned Schwenkter, M.D., as well as the managers of the clinical and support units, was the driving force behind this managed change program.

Interpreting the Grid. Figures 2, 3, 4, and 5 provide data from Elizabethtown University Hospital's Healthcare Organization Assessment Survey. Note that the initial total group score was particularly low in commitment, job satisfaction, and strength of culture (Figure 2). These scores indicate that managers and physicians at Elizabethtown Hospital did not have a clear understanding of the organization's mission, values, or vision. Because of such a pattern, it would be difficult to gain employees' trust to participate in any kind of change program.

As Figure 3 shows, Elizabethtown managers were highly motivated to perform their jobs well. However, the employees also saw the organization as not providing much in the way of recognition for hard work.

The greatest areas of disparity existed between organizational power and organizational affiliation. Managers did not view the hospital as encouraging participation in decision making or encouraging or rewarding employees to be more aggressive and to take

**Figure 2. Organizational Assessment and Development Process
Analysis Grid (Total Group).**

Influence / Value Stressed	Person	Job	Organization
Recognition			
Pre	13%	28%	16%
Post	12%	90%	72%
Accomplishment			
Pre	55%	56%	33%
Post	60%	76%	80%
Power			
Pre	42%	48%	20%
Post	38%	74%	58%
Affiliation			
Pre	100%	70%	13%
Post	100%	88%	68%

	Commitment	Satisfaction	Strength of Culture
Pre	31%	28%	2%
Post	82%	70%	80%

risks. These personal scores coupled with a low strength of culture indicated that the managers wanted to be team players and to try innovative approaches. But they were unsure about where the hospital was going and uncertain that it would welcome such initiatives.

The subgroup scores for the administration echo the total group score with one notable exception. Members of the administration had a very high commitment score. This means that although

**Figure 3. Organizational Assessment and Development Process
Analysis Grid (Administration).**

Value Stressed \ Influence	Person	Job	Organization
Recognition			
Pre	32%	40%	41%
Post	58%	96%	92%
Accomplishment			
Pre	59%	80%	74%
Post	96%	94%	98%
Power			
Pre	76%	57%	17%
Post	94%	86%	44%
Affiliation			
Pre	100%	90%	30%
Post	98%	96%	94%

	Commitment	Satisfaction	Strength of Culture
Pre	86%	53%	10%
Post	98%	96%	100%

they too were uncertain of the hospital's direction, they were dedicated to strengthening its culture and to implementing a change program. Most important, their high affiliation and medium power scores showed that they would be able to work as a team to accomplish change.

The scores of the nurse managers subgroup showed several variations from the scores of the total group (Figure 4). Nurse man-

Figure 4. Organizational Assessment and Development Process
Analysis Grid (Nursing).

Value Stressed \ Influence	Person	Job	Organization
Recognition			
Pre	84%	26%	2%
Post	70%	94%	88%
Accomplishment			
Pre	56%	19%	18%
Post	40%	82%	90%
Power			
Pre	94%	50%	60%
Post	60%	86%	78%
Affiliation			
Pre	96%	31%	3%
Post	100%	94%	94%

	Commitment	Satisfaction	Strength of Culture
Pre	37%	10%	2%
Post	92%	98%	88%

agers had higher personal values scores than they did job or organization scores—a typical indication of a morale problem. These
nurse managers identified very closely with their profession and not
at all with the hospital. Before nurse managers would be willing to
participate in a change program, they would have to commit themselves to trusting the hospital (understanding the pressure the hospital was under to provide quality care with shrinking resources),

**Figure 5. Organizational Assessment and Development Process
Analysis Grid (Medical Staff).**

Influence / Value Stressed	Person	Job	Organization
Recognition			
Pre	2%	43%	68%
Post	2%	100%	88%
Accomplishment			
Pre	78%	80%	71%
Post	64%	98%	58%
Power			
Pre	17%	36%	2%
Post	30%	92%	70%
Affiliation			
Pre	60%	90%	92%
Post	36%	98%	66%

	Commitment	Satisfaction	Strength of Culture
Pre	60%	81%	35%
Post	98%	100%	64%

and the hospital would have to give the nurses something they
could believe in. In contrast to the nurses, physicians showed a
better understanding of the hospital's mission and greater commitment to the hospital (Figure 5).

Using the Audits to Identify Areas for Change. The uni-
formly low strength of culture scores indicated that the first order

of business was to review all audit statements relating to strength of culture and commitment. As a result of this audit process, the administration decided that it needed to redefine the hospital's mission and values. In addition, the nurse managers looked at all audits relating to recognition, accomplishment, and affiliation, paying particular attention to such matters as teamwork, participation in management, career succession and advancement, and performance appraisal.

The structured process of staff assessment, analysis of data, and review of audits paved the way for a very successful managed change program, as shown by the high postassessment scores. The leadership process used by Jeffrey Norman and his team is described below. This same process has been used by other successful health care leaders throughout the country.

Identifying the Barriers to Strengthening Your Culture. As you move from assessment to analysis, you must challenge the mission and values of your organization, but it is its vision that becomes the centerpiece, the pivot point upon which you will make your initial judgment. Take a quick inventory of your organization as documented in financial statements or marketing plans. Do you find evidence of increased bad debt, financial disappointments in new business ventures, retention problems among subspecialists, inadequate information systems, or a weak image among local businesses?

As a next step, overlay your mission statement on these data. To what extent does a problem identified here prevent you from achieving your mission? For example, suppose that part of your mission is to generate revenue through managed-care contracts with local area employers. Suppose further that the data reveal that you have employees who are high in the intangible of affiliation but low in accomplishment? They may be able to talk about the service, but can they close the sale, as it were? It will be difficult to achieve your mission with people who value support and caring more than financial success and the development of new linkages with local businesses. There is too great a disparity between corporate values and personal values. However, if your mission is to maintain the healing tradition of a specific religious order, you may fall short with individuals who score high in power and low in affiliation.

In analyzing the fit of your mission with the values of the work force, you should address several issues:

First, to what extent do your perceived problems touch on your mission? In light of your mission, what are your real problems or challenges? What trends should you be concerned about? On which people, situations, and events should you focus your attention and assets?

Second, given the priorities identified in your mission statement, where do your people stand? Do the data show that your work force understands its role sufficiently to move the organization forward in the achievement of your mission? Or do the values profiles indicate that the organization may remain in a holding pattern or regress in the near future? To what extent is their understanding of mission an indication that they would impede achievement of your goals?

Third, as an exercise, describe what the organization would be like if it were actively achieving its mission. How would it be different? Would the work force as it currently exists be the same? How would its members need to change?

Fourth, summarize in what ways the dynamics of your work force encourage the fulfillment of your overall mission and in what ways they tend to block it.

Analyzing Your Core Values: What Drives Your Decisions?
After analyzing your mission, look at your core beliefs. What convictions underpin choices in your organization? What is seen as most important? Is it respect for life, community support, and teaching? Or is it opportunity, innovation, and excellence? After you have identified your values (the convictions that drive your decisions), examine what the data say about the values of your work force. Once again, there may be conflicts between your organization's stated values and the operating values of your work force.

In an organization that truly values caring and the dignity of the individual, people who have low affiliation scores and high power scores may face the classic problem of poor organizational fit. Why? Because if they are low in affiliation, they will probably never place much emphasis on caring for others. Therefore, people who value winning, success, and external recognition may find themselves at odds with an organization whose statement of philosophy refers to "vocation," "service," and "the noble act of caring." In analyzing values, ask these questions:

1. What are the lived values of this organization—not just those that we pay lip service to?
2. To what extent does the values profile of our work force complement or contradict our optimal organizational values profile?
3. What problems might result from a conflict in values? In contrast, what could be achieved if the values of the organization meshed with those of the work force?
4. If a values conflict is uncovered, what are the options for dealing with it?

One CEO wanted to reinforce his organization's role in making the community a better place in which to live. Unfortunately, some of the managers were motivated exclusively by external rewards and seldom spoke of "healing," "charity," or "vocation." Using a similar reward system for all managers produced rebellious, cynical subgroups and decreased motivation and productivity. No matter how hard this CEO tried, an affiliative mission whose core values were healing and caring made no impression on managers who, in philosophy and practice, would have felt right at home with Machiavelli.

At the present time, this CEO is still struggling to find a solution to the problem. Should he terminate the competent, but mercenary managers and hire more caring replacements? Is there any hope of getting his managers to "meld into" the organization's mission and value system? Ultimately, he may have to compromise and use different forms of motivation on different managers, depending on their personal values profiles. One thing is certain: In designing any system, this CEO must always keep his mission in mind. Leaders never design the mission around the people; rather, they build a team to support the mission. The ship's captain doesn't ask the crew where the ship should go! If the crew doesn't want to go to the ship's destination, then they should leave the ship.

Creating the Vision: Where Are You Headed? Once you know why your organization exists and what you believe in, you can decide where you want to go. In structuring your vision, you should move through a three-step process:

First, describe the direction and goals of the organization. Choose only a direction that relates to your mission and value system. This direction may involve a number of categories:

- *Social:* demographics; escalating patient expectations; changing values about work and family; growth of the elderly population; changes in ethnic composition.
- *Technological:* information systems; decision support systems; artificial intelligence; pharmaceutical advances; medical developments; preventive strategies; ethical issues; reimbursement.
- *Economic:* regulation of charges; determination of services and sites; establishment of payment procedures; influence of health manpower tort reform.
- *Environmental:* changes in diet; smoking; teenage pregnancy; alcohol and substance abuse; AIDS; homelessness; the uninsured; the aging.
- *Manpower:* malpractice; payment limitations and variations; cost of medical education; supply and retention of nurses and allied health professionals.

Second, examine the implications of your vision. What does the vision mean? What is its potential impact? How might this vision influence physicians, trustees, nurses, and allied health professionals? What does it mean for your organization in terms of human resources, finance, facilities, programs and services, marketing, planning, governance, and community relations? Gauge the systemic impact of your vision on various groups within the hospital as well as on current divisions, departments, functions, or special constituencies. In pursuing this line of argument, ask questions such as these:

- *Social:* What will be the impact on health care of the increased number of women working outside the home? How could the aging of the baby-boom generation affect your approach to wellness and prevention of disease? How might an increase in AIDS cases affect your hospital?

- *Economic/public policy:* What will be the impact of changes in methods of reimbursement? How might the system impact patient discharge, limitation of care to the severely ill, or outpatient services? Will your hospital one day be forced to close its doors?
- *Technological:* Are you able to afford new technologies? What technologies should be given priority? How much will technology reduce the cost of health care? How much will it increase costs? Given your mission and service area, what technologies will be necessary? How will reimbursement impact your purchase and use of technology?
- *Manpower:* How will the growing shortage of nurses and allied health professionals impact you? Will you be able to attract primary care physicians and specialists to your organization and area?

Third, discuss the strategic and tactical plans needed to achieve your vision. What are the broad strategies that you plan to pursue? For example:

- *Technological:* Are you abreast of developments in technology as well as changing reimbursement patterns? Have you educated your public about technological developments and dilemmas?
- *Social:* Do you offer services adapted to the needs of working women, the aged, teenage mothers, those who are seriously overweight, the drug and alcohol addicted?
- *Manpower:* How can we restructure the environment to give nurses and ancillary personnel more professional responsibilities and more opportunities to advance?
- *Economic:* Have you enhanced efficiency (in response to declining reimbursement) through innovative staffing, techniques, new purchasing methods, and the establishment of alternative sites?

Exhibit 3 is an exercise that will help you to develop your vision statement.

Exhibit 3. Exercise: Creating a Vision Statement.

This exercise is designed to help you articulate your vision for your department, division, or organization. A vision has several characteristics. Discuss each one separately before writing out a vision statement.

Visions are statements of destination, so they are forward looking. How far into the future are you able to look?

Visions are conceptualizations of hopes for the future. they state what the end results should look like. Using words and phrases, describe your desired end result.

Visions express a sense of the possible, not the probable. They are expressions of the ideal, the standard of excellence. Describe what you want to have happen (not what you think will happen) in your vision.

Visions are unique: they set you apart from everyone else. This singularity fosters commitment. Describe how your vision would set you apart from others.

The job of the leader is to communicate his or her vision to others and to gain their commitment to that vision. Review your previous statements and then write a vision statement in twenty-five words or less.

If you feel really ambitious, try to reduce this statement to a ten-word sentence.

Chapter Eight

Action:
Implementing Successful Changes

It is finally done: The organization has been assessed. Its strengths and weaknesses have been analyzed on the basis of core values. Now it is time to take action. The action plan specifies what will be done, who will be responsible for its various components, and how rapidly the plan will move forward. It is, of course, the organization's culture that must structure the plan of action, including such highly important factors as the timing, style, and tone of the plan.

Let us think here of an executive who is overstressed because of the number of changes—and the pace of change—in her hospital. For years she has felt her predicament worsen and constantly recites to herself a litany of potential perils and risks. She has endured self-righteous lectures by well-intentioned friends on the human value of her work environment. But the question still remains: What can she do about the need for change? Part of the answer rests in her ability to look inward and ask herself fundamental if difficult questions: Who am I—as a person and as a professional? What am I expected to accomplish and will the accelerating pace of change prevent me from achieving my goals? The way she chooses to define her mission, values, and vision will determine her ability to cope with change and her methods for doing so.

Reasonable Goals

If they are to act, leaders must operationalize culture by translating the organization's mission into practical concerns: What is possible? What is realistic? What will work? What resources—time, talent, energy, and money—will be needed to make this action plan work?

If the organization is already troubled by dysfunctional individuals, there are several deceptively simple options available to the leader. He can (1) terminate the current band of organizational outlaws and find appropriate replacements, (2) introduce strategies to change their behavior, or (3) identify new strategies to motivate them to become more productive.

In choosing among these options, the leader must again consider the organization's culture and ask himself: What are we trying to achieve? What is our purpose? Then, he must determine if individuals will contribute constructively to achieve the mission or are more likely to sabotage its fulfillment. If the latter outcome is probable, only two courses of action are open to him: Change the culture or change the people.

Hard-core, traditional executives may take what looks like the easy way out and move swiftly toward termination and replacement of organizational renegades. But leaders who weather the assessment and analysis process often discover that their problems are more complex than they had anticipated and not easily resolved by eliminating people. Why? Because in the course of determining what motivates people to work, leaders often discover that the problem is the product of weak relationships among employees, their jobs, and the organization.

For example, a health care executive who completes the assessment and analysis process may discover that she has fifty senior and middle managers who are more motivated by affiliation and caring than by achievement. At about the same time, the organization reaffirms that "productivity is our number one priority." Will well-meaning, good-hearted people be effective in this organization? Is it possible to motivate them to place less emphasis on caring and more on achievement? Can their jobs be restructured to blend caring with achievement? Or should the organization do an about-face and boldly assert, "Caring is our number one priority?"

Organizations face similar pressures when external events force a change in culture. A flamboyant CEO of a Midwest community hospital put together a hard-driving management team composed of executives who were primarily motivated by recognition and money. In the wake of prospective payment and greatly increased competition, however, the organization has begun to cut back its services and staff and has redefined its mission to state, "We're going to do more with less and stress high quality and consumer satisfaction." Is it any wonder that a management group accustomed to basking in the limelight and seeing tangible rewards in its paychecks would start to feel confused, angry, and demoralized? What, then, can the CEO do? Should he try to transform his managers and persuade them to accept the wisdom of "small is beautiful?" Should he try to discover other, nontraditional ways to provide recognition and compensation? Or should he do another about-face and change the newly articulated mission and values?

The CEO described above faces a typical crisis of executive action. Where are we going? What can we do? What is possible, realistic, and workable? How serious is this "illness"? Will antibiotics be sufficient or is major surgery needed? In many cases, the executive concludes that the organization needs both. These executives find it tough to accept the reality that ambition and good intentions are no guarantee of success.

To use an analogy, it would be futile to offer someone a million dollars to grow seven feet tall, because no amount of money would help him to achieve that goal. In the same way, it is useless to offer people corner offices, leased automobiles, and expense accounts if they lack the ability to fulfill your expectations.

Leaders understand that the more you push in a direction counter to peoples' nature, the more they will rebel. Put another way, the greater the pressure to achieve the impossible, the greater the frustration. And all too often, frustration turns to aggression. The nurse may covertly attack the supervisor who again and again brings up the importance of the bottom line during an annual evaluation. The accountant may turn his mandate into a company joke by filling every memo and report with lofty phrases and euphemisms. Others may expend their energy trying to prove that change is impossible.

Too many executives believe that they can set up expectations, introduce incentives, communicate a positive attitude, and thereby get what they want. But the gospel of "stretch for success" is effective only when people can move toward a goal with their self-esteem and integrity intact. If they feel debilitated and demoralized, everyone loses—especially the organization. Communicating expectations with only limited understanding of their potentially traumatic effects on people is a form of slow-motion suicide. Leaders avoid empty rhetoric.

What, then, can leaders do? First of all, they can reduce expectations—not their vision—so that people have more time to catch up. In the meantime, they discuss expectations with other executives in comparable situations to determine if their goals are realistic and workable. Next, they can build safety nets for people so that they have the opportunity to take some risks, experiment with a new behavior or skill, and develop a sense of how they can best achieve the leader's vision in the long term. At the same time, leaders must exercise patience with people who try to change but fail the first few times. Finally, leaders can take people as far as they are able to go and give them every opportunity to succeed. They accept the reality that some will not succeed and that they may have to be replaced.

Tell a person who wants to begin a modest exercise program to get ready to run a twenty-six mile marathon in eight months and she may end up hating you. Even worse, she may grow so discouraged she will do nothing. But give that same person a specific, achievable goal such as walking for a half-hour four times a week, and she may thank you for getting her started on the road to better health.

Keep the goal within reach, and your followers will build a strong culture based on successful achievement of small, vision-specific tasks.

In moving from assessment to analysis to action, leaders identify the barriers to achieving the organization's vision. How formidable are the barriers? Can they be eliminated? Are there people who will be able to effect the change? What do they need in order to be successful? If the barrier is too great for the present staff members to surmount, the leader has the choice of changing his expectations or changing his people. To stand stoically by and do nothing is folly. Everyone will grow frustrated and angry, and the organization will falter in the process.

Identifying Essential Change Elements

Once an executive decides that her current team can fulfill the organization's mission, are prepared to accept its values, and can achieve its vision, she is ready to initiate the change process by identifying the essential change elements. Essential change elements ask the key question: To fulfill our mission in the context of our values and to achieve our vision, what do we need to change?

As an exercise, people can be asked to list all the barriers to achieving the vision and describe how difficult it will be to remove each of them. As a starting point, they may give special attention to specific behaviors and policies, focusing on the question, What behaviors and policies detract from or enhance staff performance? At one hospital, for example, every expenditure above $100 once required approval by a vice-president. Now, because essential change elements have been identified, anyone at the managerial level and above can approve expenditures up to $5,000. If managers make a mistake or commit an error in judgment, they are held accountable for their decisions. But they feel more empowered as managers.

The goal of all leadership is to produce a self-managed work force. Everything in the organization should be reviewed with the aim of encouraging employees to think like responsible adults rather than like children or interchangeable parts of a machine. Consider the issue of time. If people are burdened—especially professional-level staff—with rigid time and attendance requirements, they will very likely become clock-watchers. They will perform assigned tasks and functions within the specified hours and then bolt for the door. If the goal is to stimulate people to move faster and farther than ever before, then the focus should be put on achieving goals. If the goal is quality and high performance and not discipline and conformity, then people must be free from the often oppressive shackles of time.

In seeking out the essential change elements of the organization, you should scrutinize several areas: recruitment, employment and hiring, orientation, communication, recognition, compensation, incentives, and termination procedures. Certain questions should be asked about each of these areas: What is it about the way we hire, orient, communicate with, or reward people that stands in the way of achieving our vision? What factors can we eliminate to decrease destructive, internal competition and help people feel more valued and appreciated.

In conducting this inquiry, you should take a realistic approach. For example, it is a myth that removing one bad apple or even an entire bag of apples will automatically alleviate or cure a problem. In spite of extensive terminations or a major restructuring, the problem may be so deeply embedded in the job or organization that not even wholesale firings or a major restructuring will solve it.

Although it may be beyond a leader's power to convert or otherwise transform individuals and groups, organizational systems can be altered. If people have felt oppressed, victimized, or intimidated by these systems, even minor adjustments may cause them to behave differently.

In addition to reviewing the areas listed above, a leader who takes time to critique technologies may find that they interfere with achieving his vision. In recent years, many a CEO, CIO, and an heir apparent, the CTO (chief technology officer), have fallen prey to the seductive lure of new equipment. Compelled to acquire the newest and the best, they often ignore or minimize the significance of the people who will use it. At issue are several questions: How can the organization make better decisions about technology? Who should be involved in the decision-making process and according to what criteria should acquisitions be made? How should new technologies be monitored and evaluated?

As a leader brings people together to discuss the organization's essential change elements, he returns once again to its mission, values, and vision. He reviews the group's perceptions and tries to build a consensus by addressing questions such as these: Is this the business purpose we all feel committed to? Are these the core convictions that are important to us? Is this the direction in which we want to go?

Your Role in the Change Process

The following guidelines may help you when introducing a change process:

- Understand that there are no quick fixes when it comes to most human behavior. Change takes time—sometimes months, even years. Exercise patience and compassion, but know when to cut losses if the situation seems hopeless.
- Remember that no one can do everything—no matter how noble his intentions or how strong his expectations of himself.
- Take time to document the difference between your vision of the organization and current realities. Once people understand the gap, they will become more sensitive to what it will take to move forward.

Once the essential change elements have been established, people will be eager to move ahead. You can then ask this series of questions:

- What is stopping us?
- What aspects of the organization must be changed?
- What aspects must be repaired or rectified?
- What aspects must be eliminated?
- What elements must be added?

Consider the example of the woman who needs to lose fifty pounds. She understands why she should lose weight and looks forward to increased energy, health, and attractiveness. She can envision herself as a more buoyant and active person with a lower cholesterol count. Her first question is important: What is it about the way I live my life that must be changed? As a start, she will have to stop eating 650-calorie blueberry muffins for breakfast and going out for pitchers of beer after work.

The next question is even more critical: Now that I know what must be changed, how do I do it? At breakfast, she will probably substitute low-calorie cereal, fruit, and skim milk for muffins. Diet soft drinks and mineral water will become the staples of her after-work get-togethers. In addition, she will "snack-proof" her refrigerator by filling it with low-calorie alternatives; she will avoid social occasions where she is likely to eat high calorie foods; she will even take care not to drive by her favorite fast-food haunts.

Aside from substituting behaviors, she will also add new elements to her life: a half-hour, four-times-a-week exercise program, a daily twenty-minute meditation session to control stress, and a regular class in pen-and-ink drawing to provide a diversion from eating.

Organizations must take a similar approach. Identification of barriers that must be reduced or eliminated will produce several common themes that can then be translated into essential change elements. These elements are critical to strengthening the organization's culture.

In many cases, it is intangible factors such as trust, respect, concern, and pride that will be identified. Typically, people will make statements like these: "We want to feel better about working here." "We want to relate better to co-workers." "We want to spend less time gossiping and bickering." As a group identifies essential change elements, it asks this question about each one: Is this element critical to strengthening our culture?

Guidelines for Change

Once the organization's vision has been articulated, the team can ask the following questions: What changes must be made around here? What needs to be done to make this vision come true? What barriers must be destroyed, accepted, or lowered if we are to achieve our vision and fulfill our mission? What *must* change?

Decisions on these essential change elements must be rooted in the organization's culture. If the culture is weak, a culture enhancement process may be needed. The first step here would be to refer back to the organization's mission and values. When a leader shouts, "Charge that hill," she doesn't want followers who respond,

"Sorry, but we don't think the organization is worth it." People need to be inspired to follow in the direction that the leader has set.

In identifying essential change elements, a leader may want to follow this advice:

1. Make sure the entire team understands where the organization is headed.

2. Engage team members in a process to reach consensus on the essential change elements—what it will take for the organization to succeed and what barriers presently exist that inhibit achievement of the vision.

3. Reach agreement on how the group will identify the essential change elements. Take the time to explain the entire process and its expected outcomes before beginning.

4. Begin with the mission statement as already developed and approved. If the group's focus begins to waver, remind its members of the organization's vision.

5. Reinforce the notion that all essential change elements must be seen as barriers to achievement of the vision.

6. Request that team members abide by certain guidelines: Everyone must contribute to the process; every idea, no matter how outrageous, deserves a hearing; there should be no challenging, criticizing, or ridiculing of ideas; and all ideas must be written down and reviewed.

7. Begin each essential change element statement with "We must . . ."

8. Focus on the organization, not on specific departments or individuals. For example, if someone declares, "We need to get rid of that loser in finance," turn the discussion to the types of behavior that must be eliminated or enhanced if the organization is to succeed. Always distinguish between people and behaviors.

9. Limit the number of essential change elements to no more than eight and no fewer than four. Consolidate essential change elements to the minimum number required to achieve your vision.

10. Devote each essential change element to a single issue.

11. Be prepared to invest three hours in the entire process.

In developing the list of essential change elements, the leader will want to move through the following five-step, 180-minute exercise (Exhibit 4) with the key members of the management team:

Exhibit 4. A Process for Identifying Essential Change Elements.

Step One:	Take thirty minutes to silently generate ideas on the following three questions: 1. What are the main issues or problems surrounding this organization? 2. What programs, services, or remedies would help us deal with these problems? 3. How can we best implement these programs or services?
Step Two:	Take forty-five minutes to complete a round-robin listing of ideas on a flip chart.
Step Three:	Take sixty minutes to ask for clarification on each idea.
Step Four:	Ask each individual to silently list and rank the ideas for thirty minutes.
Step Five:	Take fifteen minutes to discuss the ranking.

Some of the essential change elements generated by this exercise may be very broad; others may be very specific. They may range from "We need a better system of evaluating performance" to "We need to eliminate destructive gossip among department managers." Consider the following sample list of essential change elements:

*   We must invest in state-of-the-art information systems.
*   We must improve communications with the various publics that use the hospital.
*   We must enhance the organization's self-concept and self-esteem.
*   We must document our service to the community.
*   We must create mechanisms for making ethical decisions on resource allocation.
*   We must monitor, track, and motivate our work force.
*   We must learn to serve an ethnically diverse population.

If the essential change elements are identified by a group, they must be accepted without evaluation. At that point, the group will be ready for a more detailed analysis of the elements:

1. Why should we change? Briefly restate the reasons for change. How will the organization benefit from this change? In what ways will things improve?

2. How should we change? Briefly identify a broad approach for addressing each essential change element. For example:

Essential Change Element	*Strategy*
Track motivation of work force	Repeat annual assessment
Support ethnic diversity	Identify peoples' customs and life-styles
Improve communication	Provide education and better technology
Communicate service	Develop new linkages

3. How will we know that we have achieved our vision? Identify the criteria by which team members will evaluate their success. For example:

Essential Change Elements	*Criteria*
Track motivation	Fewer complaints, less sabotage
Ethnic diversity	Better responses from opinion leaders
Improve communication	Quicker response times
Communicate service	Strong positive responses to customer satisfaction surveys

From the essential change elements will come a small number of specific behaviors that will in turn become the focus of performance. These behaviors can be classified according to one of two systems:

System 1

People: Build more management depth in professional service. Strengthen the management skills of nurses.

Systems: Develop an approach to termination that provides for successful outplacement. Connect incentive systems to achievement of the organization's vision.

Policies: Redefine leave policies to allow for management sabbaticals. Change time and attendance policies to accommodate varied work styles.

Procedures: Eliminate requisition of office supplies from central supply. Permit individual managers to make decisions concerning the use of express mail or facsimile transmittal without supervisor approval.

System 2

Recognition: Provide service awards to employees who embody organizational values. Involve family members in more organizational events.

Achievement: Develop organizationwide systems to ensure quality of service. Enhance programs for the elderly population.

Power: Increase the organization's visibility in the local and national media. Develop stronger relationships with legislators and business groups.

Affiliation: Offer employees a nonpunitive vehicle for discussing complaints, potential problems, and grievances. Increase involvement by community members on committees and special advisory councils.

People must take care not to position essential change elements along divisional or professional lines and should avoid discussions that chronicle the faults and foibles of physicians, trustees, managers, dieticians, or any other professional group. Instead, they need to keep the focus on systemic changes that will reinvigorate the entire organization.

By concentrating on a few specific essential change elements, managers can make a concerted effort to implement these behaviors throughout the organization. The essential change elements are derived from the analysis of barriers to achieving the organization's vision. The implementation of these behaviors will result in a reduction of the barriers and a strengthening of the culture.

Turning Essential Change Elements into Action

Once the essential change elements have been identified and translated into specific behaviors, they can be implemented by managers throughout the organization. The next step is to turn once again to a consideration of the organization's mission, values, and vision. For example, if the core organizational values include justice, quality, fairness, and respect for the individual, then the leader must determine whether those values are in fact addressed by the essential change elements. If not, then perhaps the organization will simply spin its wheels as it attempts to change and will never achieve its vision.

Moving into action demands performance plans—specific events and checkpoints that detail who does what, when, where, and how. After each manager develops an individual performance plan for each behavior, he or she must describe how things will be different once changes have been made.

In the midst of the change process, executives often realize the wisdom of the saying "Little things mean a lot." Suppose the essential change element is to enhance recognition, and the leader will have achieved success when people say thank you more often. Unfortunately, many executives scoff at change on this seemingly basic level. "Of course, I appreciate my people," they claim. "I thank them all the time." To test the validity of this kind of assertion, one executive kept a one-day tally of his thank you behavior. To his surprise, at 4:00 P.M., he began to say thank you deliberately—just to amass a respectable score. Although he appreciated peoples' contributions, saying thank you simply was not in his repertoire of behavior. On the basis of one insight, that executive now relates to colleagues and co-workers in a dramatically different way.

This executive's response was only one example of how his organization had to change from the top down. If that organization wanted to make the value of recognition come alive, there would be nothing more powerful, more easy, or less expensive than having that executive—and others like him—say, "Thanks a lot for your help. I really appreciate the way you took care of things for me."

For executives, the lesson is clear. They must learn to appreciate the power of the individual. If 1,900 employees changed one thing about their behavior that would help the organization fulfill its mission and achieve its vision, that would mean 1,900 changes. Massive consequences would be generated. Go a little further. If each of those individuals changed one behavior each quarter, almost 8,000 changes a year would be produced.

The leader's role is to make positive, vision-focused change a routine event for everyone in the organization. To reinforce the importance of such change, people need to be asked to regularly record or note positive behaviors. What effect did the change have on their behavior? What was the impact of the change on others? How will the new behavior change their relationships? Most importantly, they need to share with others the ways in which they have changed. In one hospital, an executive described how he had changed his strategy for terminating an employee. In previous years, he often forced employees to resign through harassment and intimidation. Just as often, however, the employee stayed around long enough to sabotage projects and spread resentment. After practicing a simple three-step process—define, discipline, and discharge—the executive reported than he could compassionately terminate an employee and avoid the pain of interpersonal conflict.

For a leader, the strategy for implementing organizational change is as follows:

First, recommend ways for taking note of behavioral improvements. This might be as simple as a tally in a notebook or a daily entry in a work diary.

Second, create ways for employees to share their change experiences with others. At the beginning of each major meeting, forum, retreat, or professional development program, refer back to the organization's mission, values, and vision to provide a context for any changes that may be discussed.

Third, share personal change experiences, especially those that relate to the organization's mission, vision, and values. It takes courage for an executive to admit before a group, "I went out of my way to help a patient with a problem today. Before we started this process of looking at who we are and where we are headed, I would have blamed someone else for the problem or passed the buck. But today, I took a small part of my day to help someone who really needed it."

Last, give employees the support they need to make changes. If this requires development of a particular skill, then make sure that the appropriate program is instituted. It is futile to encourage people to be innovative if they do not have the necessary cognitive and behavioral skills.

To begin the change process, people must be challenged to share at least one thing they plan to change each week for a series of weeks. Then, people must begin the process within twenty-four hours of the initial meeting.

In an effective organization, everyone—from the chairman of the board to the dietary services worker—has made a commitment to changing in ways that will help the organization achieve its vision. Just as the would-be dieter can make commitment to lose four ounces a day, so can people within an organization achieve success by committing themselves to making one small change and then repeating it over and over again.

Therein lies the difference between a manager and a leader. In their zeal to change things as quickly as possible, managers often autocratically force solutions on others. Leaders, in contrast, empower people to solve their own problems by giving them realistic goals and the confidence and power to attain them. Becoming obsessed with detail and data, managers sometimes begin to act like lords of the manor. But leaders have the courage to share their continual struggle to overcome their own weaknesses. But they also know that, no matter what, they will survive, and they realize that genuine power comes from empowering others, not withholding power.

Above all, leaders are willing to confront reality. Unlike the monarch in the emperor's new clothes, they will never self-righteously parade through the streets of town while their followers cheer in blind adulation. Nor will they imitate the Queen of Hearts in *Alice in Wonderland* and rampage through the hallways screaming "Off with their heads" at the slightest sign of deviant behavior.

Unfortunately, however, the Queen of Hearts' vindictive scenario is still practiced in too many organizations. One CEO has earned the nickname "the Terminator" because of the way she treats employees who dare to question her authority. Before meetings, managers must print their questions on blank cards and hand them to an associate who screens them lest the CEO be embarrassed by any "stupid" or "inappropriate" queries. Needless to say, few bold, innovative, or aggressive managers stay longer than a year.

The effective CEO, in contrast, creates a conflict-free environment where everyone in the organization—from the president of the medical staff to the laboratory technician—feels liberated to think and dream. An unwritten rule undergirds every action: "This is a safe place to work. I can offer criticism and suggest better ways for doing things with no fear of reprisal. No one can hurt me for being honest and direct in helping the organization fulfill its mission."

Above all, the leader must lead the change process by example. One of the most demoralizing experiences for members of an organization is to hear a CEO say, "It's your problem; you fix it." Sometimes employees are not even aware of the problem, let alone of the most appropriate solution to it.

To be effective, senior management must lead through modeling and be willing to share—on a highly personal level—their difficulties in grappling with change and experimenting with new behaviors. A model CEO said at a staff meeting, "I'm struggling with these economic demands. We're successful now, but I want you to know that it's not easy. I came into health care because I wanted to help people, and now I spend most of my time looking at financial forecasts. But I've decided to limit my financial planning to the afternoons and use my mornings for creative work. I'm going to work on human capital as hard as I work on financial capital. What do you plan to do?"

As a leader works through the change process, she must keep the focus on the barriers to achieving the organization's vision and not on day-to-day problems. If she focuses on problems, she may contract a near-fatal case of "analysis paralysis." When the focus is on barriers, there is only one issue to pose: "Here's the barrier. Are we going to reduce it, eliminate it, or accept it?"

In fact, once people know where they are headed, they can deal with almost any barrier that stands in their way. Like the crew of a ship, they will never stray from their ultimate destination simply because they run into bad weather. Instead, they will decide—as a team—whether to change course or ride out the storm. Rather than fretting about the fate that might befall them, they will focus on home port and their reason for going to sea in the first place.

Organizations are much the same. If senior management sets a negative example through an obsession with finances, the organization probably will never build a strong bottom line. On the other hand, if the CEO focuses on mission, vision, and values, financial disaster will become almost impossible because the organization will have a strong, committed work team.

The key to executive leadership in health care is to keep employees focused on the organization's mission, vision, and value system. Decisions are made on the basis of this mission, vision, and system, and are then implemented. People will not lose their bearings because the leader will be present to remind them of their goal. And even if they encounter barriers, the leader will have built enough momentum to carry them over the rough spots. When it comes to executing change, leaders are in the driver's seat. The choices they make as organizational role models will affect every person in the organization. Remember, executives who are *caring, engaging,* and *open* will create an organization filled with people who are *committed, enthusiastic,* and *ready to seize opportunities.*

Focusing on the Target

By way of conclusion, let us refer back to the Elizabethtown University Hospital Rehabilitation Center change process discussed in the previous chapter. In that case, managers wanted to know at the very start what their new culture would be. When they discovered that significant changes were required, they began to put up considerable resistance.

The first step in the managed change process, then, was to overcome this resistance. Because the managers had high affiliation scores, it was decided to group them into teams as part of the change strategy. An alliance among the administrator, medical staff director, the new director of nursing, and the director of finance was built, and this alliance was then used to support other team activities. Two ad hoc committees were also created. One was a transition committee used to bridge the gap from old to new. The second was a new-product committee that was charged with investigating new sources of revenue. The hospital also built a management team that focused on the mission, values, and vision of the new culture and identified skills that would be needed to strengthen the financial condition of the hospital. These skills included the business of health care, finance for nonfinancial planners, and marketing.

Did the assessment, analysis, and subsequent change program make a difference? With implementation of the change program as the only major variable, the hospital went from an operating loss of 31 cents per dollar in the first half of one year to a gain of 3.2 cents in the first quarter of the next. Committed, inspired followers produce effective organizations.

PART THREE

Ensuring Organizational Vitality

Chapter Nine

Successfully Managing the Dynamics of Change

Leaders continually focus on what it takes to strengthen an organization's culture. Leadership makes it possible to create and sustain a strong culture. If a leader has true followers, he will be able to answer yes to the following questions: Do employees believe in the core values that underpin the organization? Are they committed to the direction of the organization—its vision? Do they believe in the organization's purpose—its mission?

Creating and sustaining a strong culture means that the leader defines and communicates mission, vision, and values as often as possible and through as many vehicles as possible. It means that the leader is the master storyteller and "network anchorperson" for the organization's identity, direction, and beliefs.

Another important aspect of culture is its spirit. Although often lacking a visible presence, a strong culture is felt and experienced by the people who are a part of it. Diverse personalities and types may populate a given cultural landscape, but everyone unites around a single core. In a strong culture, organizational commitment and job satisfaction run high. And, as people increasingly identify themselves with the organization, they become part of its elusive magic and spirit.

Problems Versus Conflicts

Even though people may be happy with their work, the work force is never problem free. What distinguishes a strong culture is the attitude that people take toward problems. Rather than allowing problems to defeat and demoralize them, individuals in strong cultures come to understand that problems are a part of life. When a problem arises, they simply say, "Here's what we're facing. How can we solve it in the context of our mission, vision, and values?" Instead of rushing to adopt the latest management trend, they faithfully turn to their context—their values and vision—to relieve the pressure of the moment.

Weak organizational cultures exacerbate problems because people lack a context in which to make decisions. Not having an overall focus, individuals turn to their personal value systems for direction. A leader of a strong culture will forge diverse personal values into one culture, thereby channeling everyone's energy toward solving problems. In a weak culture, however, people have nothing to believe in but themselves. Compelled to use their own values as a basis for making decisions, they are inclined to say, You haven't given me anything to believe in, so I'm going to make decisions in my own best interests.

In summary, although people always turn to values when making decisions, leaders of strong cultures help people arrive at decisions in the context of a corporate value system that is larger than the individual or any group of individuals. Weak cultures, in contrast, force people to think of themselves first.

A problem can be viewed as an opportunity or as a source of conflict. Conflict thrives in weak cultures. Although people may appear to be arguing about how to solve a problem, their arguments usually reflect a lack of focus. Witnessing these conflicts, managers resort to traditional conflict resolution techniques when they should be building a permanent context for solving problems and avoiding conflicts. Solving problems and resolving conflicts involve very different dynamics.

At some point during the evolution of a problem, people in weak cultures make the unconscious decision to turn a problem into a conflict. For example, to address the issue of nurse recruitment and retention, an organization may decide to increase the pay of nurses by 15 percent. Understandably, pharmacists, physical therapists, occupational therapists, and ancillaries grow bitter and resentful at the special treatment accorded to nurses. They begin to think only of personal survival.

In a strong culture, however, the leader focuses on the broad issue of delivering care: What kind of culture, belief system, and vision do we have? How can we work together to deliver health care? Other than nurses, who are the professionals who deliver health care, and how can we bring them together to solve this problem? What are nurses doing now that could be done successfully by others?

If the culture is strong, a leader can position a problem in the context of an organization's vision and vlaues. But if the culture is weak, he will be more inclined to examine a problem in isolation. Instead of looking at the problem in context, he may try to push it to the side or find someone to blame, or he may try to make a few repairs. Leaders solve problems and avoid conflicts.

Role Modeling

The most powerful weapon in building a strong corporate culture is a leader who can function as a role model. Members of the work force—potential followers—will put more credence and faith in her behavior than in speeches, memos, or the glowing message at the front of the annual report. What she does counts for much more than what she says. People *listen* to behavior.

The critical intangible that binds a strong culture is trust. Trust results from consistent, reliable, and predictable behavior on the part of leaders. The work force must have faith that the leader will continually say and do the right thing for the organization. Once he says one thing and does another, that bond of trust is broken—not to be easily or quickly repaired. Trust is very hard to develop and easy to weaken, and it must be earned every day. Titles are given, trust is earned.

A CEO of a large hospital may talk a good line about productivity and organizational excellence, but the work force knows that he invariably arrives each morning after 9:30 A.M., takes extended lunches, and then proceeds to scream at people for not getting things done. He pontificates about mission, spouts the latest management lingo, and has all the right executive props and accouterments, but his words mean nothing to the work force because he is unable to back up his rhetoric with action. His behavior angers and offends the work force and will continue to erode its trust and reduce its productivity.

Communicating Culture Through Symbols

Along with behavior and words, symbols and icons can take on an almost mystical significance in organizations. A leader who understands the power of symbols splashes the corporate logo on everything from the cafeteria to the boardroom. Through slogans and mottoes, he continually reminds the work force of the organization's purpose, direction, and value system.

Although words are necessary and important, symbols are also needed to fuse together a population. When people look at the American flag, they feel a rush of emotions because the flag expresses their deepest feelings about freedom, democracy, and justice. This phenomenon also occurs in organizations: Workers feel pride and personal satisfaction when they see a remodeled lobby, a beautiful playroom in the pediatrics department, or a new atrium in a skilled nursing care facility. These are physical representations of their values.

Just as there must be a direct correlation between words and behavior, so there must be a direct correlation between symbols and behavior. Although mission, vision, and values are the basic ingredients of culture, trust is the glue that holds it all together. Therefore, if people note a discrepancy between the organization's symbols and icons and its behavior, the glue weakens and the culture fractures. For example, although the United States contains many diverse cultures that sometimes resemble countries within a country, it is bound together by its ability to solve problems through the rule of law. Trust breaks down when white-collar criminals are acquitted or criminals go free. But every time the rule of law triumphs, the system is vindicated, and the bonds of trust between the people and the government are strengthened. Once trust is lost in an organization's leadership or in a nation's government, people tend to regress to selfish, turf-protecting behavior. The more distrust that exists, the more people revert to their personal value systems to make decisions and the more they resist anyone who tries to interfere with or even question their value systems.

What, then, is the answer? If a leader is strong, she communicates the mission, vision, and values of the organization with consistency, accuracy, and immediacy. She does not allow wounds to fester and emotions to run over. Instead, she tackles problems immediately, clarifies their meaning, and helps people work toward solutions by building a context that is consistent with the organization's mission, vision, and values.

Managing Change

Change is inevitable in the field of health care. There is no way to escape it. Moreover, the rate of change will continue to accelerate. Despite these realities, many health care executives choose to deny the dynamics of change, cloaking themselves in dangerous myths that offer little more than temporary relief from reality. Consider the popularity of the following beliefs:

Change just happens; it can't be managed. Typical reactions include: "What happens, happens. There's nothing we can do about it." "Let's wait and see what happens. We don't know what's going to happen until it happens, so let's not worry about it." "What will be, will be."

Change can be prevented or postponed through good intentions and hard work. Standard responses are: "Things always turn out for the best." "It will all work out." "Let's just continue doing what we've always done." "If it's worked for this long, it ought to keep on working." "What was good enough for us five years ago is good enough today."

Change is uniform: "It's going to turn this country upside down." "If it happened to them, it could happen to us." "Everyone will be hurt—there is nothing we can do!" But you will not hear leaders echoing these popular myths. Leaders take a broad view of the environment and then act boldly to anticipate, manage, and direct change.

Likewise, the character of the health care industry demands that organizations have infrastructures that can absorb the shocks that will inevitably hit them. Several years ago, the head of a national health maintenance organization was on the cover of an industry news magazine. Shortly after, the company went into bankruptcy. No matter how dazzling a business success story or how meteoric someone's rise to prominence, everyone is vulnerable to change.

Developing effective responses to change requires, however, that a leader understand the three basic types of change: developmental change, traumatic change, and managed change.

Developmental Change. This kind of change is inevitable in health care organizations. The ongoing cycle of seasons produces physical changes in the environment, and the same analogy holds true for people's bodies. No matter how well people take care of themselves, their bodies will change. To a certain extent, everyone experiences wrinkling of the skin or a loss of hair. Although one can postpone, soften, or control these changes, they can never stop or be reversed. Sooner or later, aging, like winter, will happen.

The same is true of change in organizations. The x-ray was replaced by magnetic resonance imaging, which has, in turn, been replaced by positive emission tomography. As long as resources are available for research and development, technology will expand and grow whether one chooses to invest aggressively in capital equipment, postpone purchases, or orchestrate joint ventures with other organizations.

In the same way, we can be confident that there will be continued change in legislation and regulation. In recent years, the majority of developmental changes in the health care industry resulted from prospective pricing. While it is impossible to predict the future, we can be fairly sure that no bureaucrat, with a single flourish of a magic wand, will return health care to the languor of cost-based reimbursement. It is likely that the health care industry will see increased developmental change in areas such as managed care, availability of manpower, and consumer choice.

Traumatic Change. Changes of this kind are typically viewed as more negative than developmental changes. The man who must cope with the developmental change of hair loss may also experience the trauma of a sports injury that leaves him bedridden for two weeks. Traumatic change can hit health care organizations in much the same way. Consider the following examples:

- A medical group leaves.
- The top admitter has a heart attack and dies.
- Three of the organization's top executives go to work for competitors.
- The board decides to terminate the CEO.
- A factory in the community closes, and three thousand families of childbearing age are lost.

Changes such as these can traumatize an organization, significantly affecting its ability to deliver service. On the opposite end of the spectrum, consider these changes:

- A new factory relocates to a nearby community and brings in 3,000 new families.
- A direct mail promotion of a new weight-management program attracts 500 people who want to sign up for a complementary orientation.
- The organization receives a $5 million grant to study the effects of home visitation on the length of hospital stay.

Although positive, these changes may also generate stress and physical disruption. Change of whatever kind often causes people to grow possessive of their territory, space, and roles. Even a change for the better may at first produce anxiety, frustration, and confusion.

Change within organizations must be handled in the same way as change within a family. When a family faces a change in economic status, an accident, or a residential move, for example, an adult leader usually emerges to assure the other family members that everything will be fine. The mother or father, or sometimes even an older sibling, will point to the benefits of the change and urge everyone to pull together to make things better than ever.

The same is true of organizations. If a health care organization is located in a sixty-year-old building that must be torn down and replaced with a more modern facility, employees may respond with comments such as: "It's not going to be the same." "Why are they spending money on bricks when they could be spending money on us?" "What's wrong with the old building?" "We're losing our history and traditions."

The leader of that organization must carefully explain the benefits of the change to employees, patients, and physicians. Most importantly, employees need to know that they will be able to carry out the organization's legacy for quality patient care with even greater energy and commitment in the new building. When the perception is altered from traumatic to developmental, change becomes more acceptable.

In the case of a developmental change, a leader can work systematically to mobilize the work force behind an idea. For example, if he is preparing to build a replacement facility, merge with another organization, or diversify into services for the elderly, he can develop specialized communication vehicles such as newsletters, conduct small-group information sessions, or create task forces to engage the work force in the change. Employees can be helped to "own" the change by turning developmental change into managed change.

Following are some strategies that leaders can use in dealing with developmental change:

Create a sense of excitement about the change. Discuss the change in terms of the benefits and advantages it will offer to various sectors of the organization and to the community. If possible, show that the perceived disadvantages or problems will simply be minor, routine occurrences in the change process.

Build confidence. Help the work force focus on its strengths and resources. Tell stories about how staff members successfully overcame problems and crises in the past.

Celebrate small victories and achievements. As the change progresses, share new developments with members of the work force. Describe to them how each step is contributing to achievement of the organization's vision.

Clarify roles for people in the context of the hoped-for outcome. Be prepared to say to the work force, This is your role in ensuring the success of this new program or service.

Be patient. Give the work force an opportunity to internalize the change. People need time to understand that, although they may be doing their jobs in the same ways, they can also take advantage of the new opportunities that a change will inevitably bring.

Provide forums in which people can discuss issues and ask questions. Don't rely on impersonal "happiness" surveys and complaint-driven suggestion boxes. Instead, create one-on-one sessions between executives and staff members or, at a minimum, sponsor small-group sessions. Often employees need reassurance on issues as simple as: Will my work space look the same? Will I be working with the same people? How will my job change? Am I still going to be doing the same types of projects? Work with them to create a positive vision of how they fit into the end result.

Evaluate the implications of change for the entire organization, assessing its tangible and intangible impact on each unit and subunit of the organization and even on specific individuals. Then take steps to address specific problems.

Exercise vigilance. Try to anticipate how changes may affect the organization. When changes are in the offing, focus everyone's attention on the barriers between the present state of the organization and your vision of its future.

When an organization is hit with traumatic change, there may not be time to develop consensus and build confidence. In contrast to developmental change, traumatic change is far more likely to produce strong emotions: Fear that borders on paranoia and anger that can easily escalate into rage. Productivity plummets as people try to protect themselves from further injury and hurt. In a traumatic situation such as this, a leader needs to respond quickly. In fact, this is one of the few times when acting unilaterally may be justified. Instead of waiting for a consensus to build, the leader needs to take dramatic, immediate action. People must be brought together to discuss their fears and candidly confront reality. A leader maintains control in this way: "I realize we have a significant prob-

lem here, but, together, we can save this organization and everything it means to the community. We are going to focus on some
specific outcomes, and while we may not have time to work with
everyone, we will work with as many people as needed to make this
happen."

The key difference between traumatic change and developmental change is the intensity of emotion involved and the speed
with which leaders must move to defuse or redirect the destructive
emotions generated by the former. In developmental change, a
leader can rely on systematic team building; in the case of traumatic
change, however, she needs to galvanize her team by first acknowledging the problem and then outlining a strategy in which everyone
can play a part.

Following are several strategies for grappling with traumatic
change:

- Recognize that communication is not a one-time event. Offer
  frequent progress reports and updates.
- Outline the next steps that must be taken. Let people know
  when additional information will be forthcoming, as well as the
  specific actions that the organization plans to take and how
  employees fit (or do not fit) into the plan.
- Stress positive outcomes. Let the work force know that the organization will survive, because "we're a team."
- Make people feel valued. Stress their indispensable role in seeing the organization through the crisis.

Of course, employing these strategies is no guarantee of success. People may still blame the leader for the organization's problems. But at least they will give him some credit for acknowledging
the crisis, setting the record straight, and taking steps to turn the
situation around.

Another role of the leader is to short-circuit any attempts to
apportion blame. In a crisis one invariably hears comments such as
the following: "The doctors don't admit enough patients here."
"Physical therapy isn't out there recruiting more rehab patients."
"Accounting doesn't go after outstanding bills." "The CEO is always at meetings—she doesn't care about us."

As long as failure is another person's responsibility, members of the work force can continue to feel absolved from all blame. Hence, the leader must persuade the work force to focus on the problem, not on one another's shortcomings: "It really doesn't matter whose fault it is. This organization is in serious trouble and unless we take action—and 'we' includes everyone from physicians to accounting clerks to dietary services workers—we may not be here in another six months. Our choice is clear: Do we spend the next six months figuring out how to downsize and do outplacement, or do we pull together to save this organization as we know it? It's your choice."

It takes courage to deliver such an ultimatum. It is easy to lead during growth periods. It is very hard to lead during times of shrinking resources. People who have shaped their identity by chronically blaming others may even look upon such a leader as a traitor to the organization. But until people accept their role in solving the organization's problems, there will be little hope for that organization. Staff members must accept that their choices are to lead, follow, or get out of the way. Complaining is *not* a choice!

In a number of successful turnarounds in the past ten years, executives were apparently able to perform a kind of organizational jujitsu; that is, they used the negative energy of the work force to shape things up. But this is a tricky and dangerous feat. The safer, more appropriate role of the leader is to neutralize destructive behavior and to create a context in which people can work to save the organization. More specifically, in addressing traumatic change, a leader's role is to give the work force permission to risk short-term failure to achieve long-term success.

Managed Change. The third kind of change is managed change. Developmental and traumatic change "fixes" the past; managed change anticipates the future. Leaders draw on the strength and expertise of the work force to plan for and orchestrate change by focusing on the vision. For example, turning a sleepy 200-bed community hospital into a major referral center requires a clear vision and managed change. It might mean establishing various links with the nearby university medical center. The hospital, for example, might serve as a conduit for the medical center's open-heart cases. Certainly, there would have to be major changes in how the hospital conducts its business and how the work force perceives itself.

Managed change starts with understanding the endgame— the desired outcome. What is the organization's vision? How will the organization know when it has been successful? Articulating the desired outcome is a way of answering the question: Where am I now and where do I want to be? For example, if a hospital wants to increase its market share in cardiology by 3 percent a year for the next five years, it first needs to determine, Where are we now? If its market share is increasing at a rate of 1 percent per year and the hospital wants to increase that rate by another two percentage points per year for five years, the next issue is to develop a strategy to accomplish this change.

Managed change is a planned process backed by a leader's ability to pose the appropriate questions about tangibles and intangibles: What is our business? Where are our best opportunities? In what direction do we want to go? What kind of staff do we need to execute the plan? And, most importantly, how do we inspire our staff members so that they will commit themselves to achieving the goal? The key to managed change is execution of well-thought-out plans and selection of the right team.

Many executives forget that change is accomplished by individuals and is therefore a highly personal experience. For example, a leader will not change much by announcing at an all-staff meeting, We're changing our market position; I expect all of you to fall in line. Managed change is not achieved by edict. Even in relatively homogeneous groups, members will have widely varying perceptions about what is important and what should or should not be changed. In the same way, although a leader can produce short-term change through the use of threats and force, he will never achieve core behavioral change that way. Simply stated, *one can change behavior only by changing peoples' minds.*

Both as individuals and as members of the organization, people need to know that a potential change matches their personal work values and will be worthwhile and valuable. Some of their most common questions are: Do I have a role in the change process? Will I be important to its success? What am I expected to do? What happens if I fail? The role of the leader is to help people know, Here's how you fit into our plans. This is what the vision means for you. For example, the obstetrics nurse who is fearful of the organization's new venture into cardiology needs to hear that the high-risk cardiology unit will focus on the congenital heart problems of children. In offering that observation, the leader may not have communicated any new evidence or data to that nurse or her colleagues—other than that they are critical in fulfilling the organization's vision. However, that is the most important communication of all.

When managing change, a leader keeps in mind that every individual is profoundly different. To effectively manage the change process, a leader needs to recognize and appreciate these differences.

In almost every situation other than those involving traumatic change, one needs to give people an opportunity to grow into the situation. People differ in their ability to process information. Some deal easily with complex ideas while others require homespun examples and extended explanations. Leaders work with people one-on-one, adapting the idea to the person rather than the other way around. The more a leader works with people in developing a strong culture, the more she will come to appreciate how unique people are. Understanding and accepting their uniqueness are among the first steps in managing change. To change the behavior of followers, as well as to manage change, a leader must first understand that not all human beings are equally bright, have equal or equivalent experiences, or are equally motivated. A parallel may be made with a glass and a bucket filled with water. Both are full, but one has more capacity than the other.

In fulfilling her role, a leader attempts to motivate people and move them through the process of assessment, analysis, and action. Her goal is a strong culture characterized by shared values, trust, and organizational commitment. If she wants to make her culture even stronger, however, she needs another skill: the ability to create strong work teams held together by trust—teams that can help her manage change in the context of her organization's mission, vision, and values.

Building Teams

Teams are used most effectively in developing new products or services, in improving quality, in evaluating and implementing new technology, in problem solving, and in quickening the decision-making process. However, Tom Peters in his book *Thriving on Chaos,* (1982, p. 364) suggests that "the power of teams is so great that it is often wise to violate apparent common sense and force a team structure on almost everything." What are the major characteristics of teams? Whether one talks about sports teams or work teams, they have several attributes in common:

- Teams have a goal.
- Teams know the rules of the game.
- Teams know how to keep score.
- Team members understand their roles in achieving the outcomes.

People are hired by an organization because they have the right combination of technical competence, skill, and experience. Unless they understand their roles or the goal of the team, however, they cannot contribute to the team's success and may, in fact, become hindrances.

Rob sold his skills as a public affairs specialist with Washington connections to a budding health care consulting firm, but lasted only six months in his newly created vice-presidential position because he never came to understand the rules of the consulting game. He failed to learn that being an entrepreneur was not compatible with long lunches, personal phone calls, and a laissez-faire attitude toward new business development. Although he was employed by an entrepreneurial company, he continued to operate by the rules of a government agency.

A leader looking at organizational team building needs to ask many of the same questions that a new coach or manager would ask:

- Who is on the team?
- What skills do they have?

- What game are they playing? Or what game do they think they are playing?
- What are the rules of this game, and is the team playing according to these rules?
- How does one keep score and ultimately win this game?
- What are the roles of the individual players? How can they support each other?

In a health care organization, an executive might ask the following questions:

- What is our target—our vision?
- How will everyone work together to reach our vision?
- What are the roles of the members of this team and of the team leader?

Playing a game involves the risk of losing, and losing often has a more disruptive effect on people in organizations than on athletes, who are used to competing day after day. When people in organizations realize that they are unable to score enough "hits" and "runs," they may refuse to deal with the situation realistically. In such situations, both a coach and a leader need to keep people focused on winning the game. Having someone go up to the batting cage and do ballet positions would be interesting, to say the least, but irrelevant to winning the baseball game. The same is true of the batter who chooses—just for fun—to run from third base to second base to first base. It would be intriguing, but unrelated to the task at hand: winning the game.

A leader needs to keep her team focused, resisting the human temptation to offer interesting but irrelevant targets. For example, people may refuse to focus on solutions by denying that a problem even exists or by taking refuge in nostalgia. Typically, they will discuss what should be rather than what is. A leader will then respond along these lines: "Yes, maybe we shouldn't have the problem, but we do. Short of divine intervention, nothing is going to change that. We need to accept that we are responsible for this problem and for trying to resolve it."

The most challenging aspect of team building is role clari-

fication. Team leaders must explain the rules of the game and clarify individual roles so that team members will understand what is
expected of them and how their participation will contribute to
success. But team members must also be involved in developing
strategies and tactics. This is what will build commitment to the
team's goal. If the strategy is to provide greater bedside care by using
care providers other than registered nurses, then the team leader
must make sure that physicians and nurses have a say in deciding
how this can be accomplished without decreasing the quality of
care. In summary, the role of a leader is to help people understand
their roles and functions on the team and give them enough focus
and direction to keep participating.

An effective leader will mobilize the medical staff by defining
the game, outlining the rules, and figuring out how everyone can
become an effective team member. The greatest contribution a
leader makes is giving people the confidence that they can succeed.
On the playing field or within organizations, leaders empower people to fulfill their roles. If players make a mistake, they may hear
about it, but they also know that they can take risks and even fail
because they have the confidence and support of the coach. The
effective leader may chew a player out with the helmet-rattling intensity of a Mike Ditka, but his last words to that player are, "All
right, now let's get back out there and try it again."

It is the presence and power of the leader that gives team
members incentive and a sense of commitment to the other players.
They will rarely, if ever, let other players down. The effective coach
or leader makes them feel as one: "This is a team. We play together.
We win together and we lose together."

Like a good coach, the effective leader can also acknowledge
personal strengths and limitations. Just as there is no way that a
conductor can play all the instruments in an orchestra, so no coach
could—or would want to—play all the positions on a team. Like
the successful coach or celebrated conductor, the effective health
care leader knows how to achieve the organization's vision by empowering each player to perform at his or her peak for the sake of
the team.

Under the tutelage of an effective coach and leader, the superstar will excel. Michael Jordan of the Chicago Bulls understands

the importance of scoring fewer points and winning the game over breaking scoring records and losing the game. Contrast that with the self-indulgent player who declares, What the rest of the team does is their own business. I'm here to score. That's how I make my money. Much to the detriment of the team, this player interprets victory and defeat from a highly selfish point of view. If the team wins, it is because he excelled; if it loses, it is because he did not get the ball enough. The effective coach or leader will know how to manage these people—either by getting rid of them, neutralizing them, or giving them enough—but not too much—rope. If tensions run high, the leader or coach will control the attitude of the players through discipline. He will lift the players high above petty gripes and egotism with the words, I don't give a damn what you think of each other; you will play this game our way or you will not be on this team.

The role of the effective leader or coach is to select the right people, empower and motivate them, and create a spirit that binds them together. A health care leader's responsibilities to teams include the following:

1. Developing an inspiring vision and then fostering team commitment to it
2. Creating a listening environment
3. Recognizing and rewarding teamwork among subordinates and others who helped the team under the leader's jurisdiction
4. Implementing team projects
5. Recruiting qualified people who are enthusiastic about team participation
6. Ensuring that all information necessary for members of a team to function successfully is made available to them
7. Ensuring that support systems are in place
8. Promoting and encouraging change, innovation, and risk taking
9. Communicating the results of team efforts across the organization
10. Reminding players that they will either win as a team or lose as a team

11.   Building a strong team and then giving its members credit for
      their efforts

      Executives must always remember that they are leaders only
if they have followers. Without committed followers, a leader cannot exist!

Chapter Ten

Increasing
Organizational
Effectiveness

The intangible side of the organizational effectiveness grid creates meaning, which is the driving force behind change and the source of organizational effectiveness (see Figure 1 in Chapter Five). The factors on the tangible side, in contrast, explain how to fulfill the organization's mission and to make it come alive for every member of the work force. Health care organizations must therefore create a balance between tangible and intangible factors.

Once the intangible underpinnings are in place—that is, once the assessment and analysis process has been completed and a managed change program has been implemented to strengthen the organization's culture—leaders can turn their attention to building the business.

This process typically begins with the formulation of strategic plans. Strategic plans have several components, including assessment of the environment, assessment of competitors, analysis of opportunities, and core and sub strategies. Assuming that a leader's plan is built on mission, values, and vision, she should have a strong grip on her business as well as the human and financial resources required to achieve the purposes of the business. Too often, however, strategic plans lack a focus on culture, the shared values of the organization. What will happen, for example, if a leader must change her organization's culture? How would she downsize the organization or diversify its operations and still maintain a strong culture and a deep commitment to the organization's values?

Developing Unit Plans

Once a leader develops a strategic plan, she can move to the creation of unit plans. The biggest criticism of strategic plans is that, like market research and doctoral theses, they usually just gather dust on the shelf. Unit plans, however, put the responsibility on managers to take the strategic plan and document and verify contributions to it. Unit plans are departmental blueprints for achieving the organization's mission, vision, and values.

Having engaged managers in the process, the leader can then ask: Can our managers implement these tactics? Do they have the cultural and technical skills to turn these plans into reality? Can they share the leadership task of strengthening the culture and communicating the staff roles? If not, then staff development is almost always the answer.

Staff Development

After communicating strategic and tactical plans, a leader turns to the professional development needs of her staff. In pinpointing gaps in knowledge and skill, she need not invest in expensive assessment tools. Instead, she lets employees and managers tell her what they need. If employees understand how their performance contributes to achieving the organization's mission, they will have no difficulty specifying their needs. Here are a few guidelines on staff development:

First, staff development should be culture based. Just as the corporate culture—mission, values, and vision—drives the organizational change process, so too should that culture drive the development of staff. In this way, staff development is closely aligned with the organization's vision and defines what skills will be necessary to achieve it.

Second, base staff development on the expressed needs of the employees. Resist the temptation to require employees to attend conferences and seminars. Instead, let the employees tell you what they need.

Third, tie staff development to the organization's tactical plans. Make sure employees understand how a structured learning experience will enhance their performance and help fulfill tactical plans.

Performance Evaluation Systems

Once employees build a base of knowledge and skills, the leader will want to explore various ways to evaluate employee performance. The routine procedures that may have been used in the past have no place here. Instead, the leader may want to focus on tactical plan performance, that is, evaluate how employees contributed to achieving the corporation's vision in the context of its values and mission.

In contrast to traditional performance appraisal systems that evoke memories of third-grade report cards, every question and topic explored in the new system must be mission driven, values based, and vision focused. For example, suppose one of an organization's core values is "respect for the individual." "Tell me," a leader might say to the director of construction and plant services, "how were you able to show respect for the patient/customer in the hospital's expansion project?"

If an organization's core values are respect, caring, commitment, and productivity, a leader might develop task forces to transform each of these values into behavior. A newly designed evaluation system would shift the focus away from "yes or no, did you do it?" to how the task was performed. *How* were employees informed about a reduction in health care benefits? When the decision was made to dissolve the marketing department, *how* was the news communicated? When community residents had to cope with construction debris, what was done to ease their inconvenience?

In this scheme, the employee who typically receives stellar reviews on fulfillment of tactical objectives could receive low ratings for betraying the organization's mission, compromising its values, or being indifferent to its vision. Consider this example: The director of finance rushes into the office and reports, I just made a

ton of money. I took that surplus cash, bought into a limited part-
nership, and we're getting a 26 percent return on equity. If a leader
were a mission-driven, values-based, and vision-focused executive,
he would have no choice but to reprimand this person if generating
revenue apart from or contrary to the mission is unacceptable behavior. Some employees may be slow to accept this view of performance. Many will retort, "Look, I'm doing my job, leave me alone."
A leader must be willing to explain, it could take weeks—even
months—as often as necessary, "Yes, I know you're doing your job,
but you have to do it in a way that enhances our mission and
achieves our vision. If you aren't supporting our purpose, what
difference does it make what you do?"

Traditionally, health care executives hired bright, well-
meaning professionals who performed tasks with little sense of
what their work meant to the organization as a whole. But this is
like asking a friend to work the rudder of a boat without telling him
the direction in which to travel. What difference does it make how
well he performs the task if he moves the boat in the wrong
direction?

Reward and Recognize Superstars

As with every previous step in managing change, a leader
must return to the organization's mission, values, and vision in
bestowing rewards and recognition. If a superstar nurse manager
ignores the mission and a B-team purchasing agent advances it,
rewards and recognition must be given to the purchasing agent if
the goal is to underscore the importance of the organization's mission and to build a team committed to that mission. People need
to have a clear notion of how they fit into the organization and they
need to see that they are contributing to something larger than
themselves.

If a leader can help people to believe in themselves and to see
the meaning in what they do, they will perform beyond his highest
expectations. But if he strips them of meaning, ridicules their beliefs, and intimidates them with fault finding, they will perform at
the rock-bottom minimum. When leaders focus on mission and not
on mistakes, people thrive and so do their health care organizations.

Discovering where a work force stands requires a thorough and sustained process of assessment, analysis, and action. Among the questions: What is the current strength of the culture? How do people perceive their jobs? What motivates employees? What leads to success, what to failure? And, finally, how can one build commitment through a closer match between person, job, and organization?

Balancing Tangibles and Intangibles

The problem facing many health care executives is that their organizations are overmanaged and underled. Managers have been directed to concentrate on profitability, market share, and productivity. Why? Partly because it is easier and less risky to deal with tangibles and partly because this is how executives have been trained. Actions taken in these spheres are likely to produce more immediate and identifiable results, and producing results is the definition of a manager. Although many health care executives still view the organization's assets as material rather than human, the axis of the industry has begun to shift. Increasingly, health care leaders and their boards resent the straightjacket of a management style driven by planning, budgeting, and control.

Although these no-nonsense, bottom-line managers meet deadlines, finish checklists, and always appear to be very, very busy, their "good management" is never enough to make a real difference for their organizations. Good management alone can never infuse an organization with spirit and energy. Good management can never build pride, trust, commitment, joy, and hope among the work force. Good management can never do what Thomas Watson did for IBM, what Ray Kroc did for McDonald's, or what Sam Walton does for Wal-Mart. Although their organizations follow the principles of well-managed organizations, they also have a "magic" that only leadership can bring.

Health care leaders of the future must be willing to play a variety of roles as they lead their organizations into the next century.

Champions of Mission. Health care leaders must champion the mission, values, and vision of the organization. They must mobilize key players to operationally define the organization's culture and then drive home its meaning to every member of the organization.

People Appraisers. Health care leaders must look at people in the same way as a jeweler looks at semiprecious stones, evaluating those who fit, those who might fit in the future, and those who no longer have a place in the organization.

Guardians of Innovation. Health care leaders must be guardians and protectors of proposed programs and services. While the bean counters pore over their spreadsheets, leaders must turn back to the basics: Will the program mesh with the organization's mission? Will it echo our value system and achieve our vision?

Cheerleaders. Rejecting lifeless traditions such as management by exception that takes no risks, health care leaders must cheer on the work force as it surges toward the finish line, must take risks, and must always be thinking about the next challenge. Instead of dwelling on blow-by-blow replays, they must liberate and empower people to stay in the game—and to win.

People for All Seasons. Health care leaders must be crusaders in their passion to celebrate the traditions and values of the past, confront the demons of the present, and lead a charge into the future. They must be the organization's source of wisdom and dreams, spinning tales of heroes and villains from days gone by. They are ships' captains, steering a course through dark, mysterious waters—always with vision—with a clear sense of where the organization is headed.

In attempting to turn themselves and their employees into good managers and nothing more, executives have overlooked the qualities that constitute true leadership. The truth is that health care executives must be both good managers and good leaders. Although leaders understand the importance of the tangibles, they know that if their organizations are to be effective, they must balance their concern for the tangibles with their concern for the intangibles. That, indeed, is the challenge of the 1990s.

Leaders must create a vision and inspire employees to achieve that vision as the first step in balancing the tangibles and intangibles. Leaders must work at building effective teams in which team members are inspired by the vision and understand their role in achieving that vision. Effective teams result in committed employees who display pride and joy in their work, feel empowered to act, and are loyal to the organization because they feel they own a piece of it.

Addressing the intangible aspects of an organization is admittedly difficult because the results of doing so are subtle and may take a long time to appear. However, if the intangibles are addressed, a major benefit is that both sides of the matrix are affected— a committed work force that shares a vision of the organization and understands its roles in achieving that vision will almost automatically produce a better bottom line. If only the tangibles are addressed, however, only the tangible side of the matrix will be affected.

Finally, a leader must be able to recruit followers, which is no easy task. It is an ongoing, demanding process, requiring consistency in actions and words and the courage to put it on the line every day in both the best and worst of times.

So, for all the leaders out there: Turn around; is anyone following?

References

Braskamp, L. A., and Maehr, M. M. "The Healthcare Organizational Assessment Survey." A Spectrum Development Program, Champaign, Ill.: MetriTech, 1986.

Maehr, M. M., and Braskamp, L. A. *The Motivation Factor: A Theory of Personal Investment.* Lexington, Mass: Heath, 1986.

Peters, T. *Thriving on Chaos.* New York: Harper and Row, 1982.

Watson, T. J. *A Business and Its Beliefs.* New York: McGraw-Hill, 1963.

Index